MY CHILD HAS WHAT?

MY CHILD HAS WHAT?

Case Studies of Common Illnesses and Problems that Five- to Twelve-Year-Old Children Face

JANET L. STAFFORD, M.D.

ILLUSTRATIONS BY PABLO RUIZ ARROYO

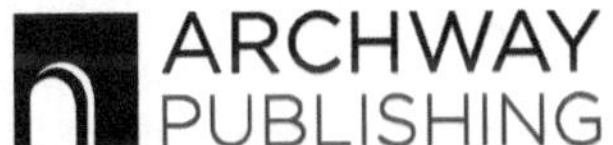

Archway Publishing books may be ordered
through booksellers or by contacting:

Archway Publishing
1663 Liberty Drive
Bloomington, IN 47403
www.archwaypublishing.com
844-669-3957

Illustrations by Pablo Ruiz Arroyo.

ISBN: 978-1-6657-0810-4 (sc)
ISBN: 978-1-6657-0808-1 (hc)
ISBN: 978-1-6657-0809-8 (e)

Library of Congress Control Number: 2021911610

Print information available on the last page.

Archway Publishing rev. date: 05/11/2022

Contents

Introduction

I was a pediatrician for decades at Kaiser Permanente Medical Group in San Francisco. Our patient population was composed of families of diverse ethnic and socioeconomic status. After retiring in my late sixties, I realized that I had been privileged to interact with many wonderful and fascinating families. I had always appreciated that the years of five to twelve are unique. In our bookstores, the sections on children are bursting with infant, preschool, and adolescent rearing advice. However, information on the crucial years of five to twelve, previously called the latency years, is sorely thin.

The period is not latent! Children in this age range are transitioning from the "fantasy-filled period" of acquiring language, fine motor skills, and social nuances of the preschooler to the "age of reason" period, when the grade-schooler around age eight understands fact versus fiction and learns the subtle aspects of honing skills and social and family interactions. I felt that I wanted to share my experiences and my input to educate families, teachers, nurses, and therapists to better understand common problems.

If this crucial period is complicated by chronic or frequent illnesses, learning differences, family turmoil, feelings of being different from peers and the child is not protected and nurtured by a caring adult in his or her life, the child may be affected physically or psychologically. Children in the age range of five to twelve are often able to mask reactions to the above complications. They do not have the breaking away beginning independence of the adolescent. The child of divorce may feel he or she has contributed to the separation and just withdraw. The child with chronic illness may either hide his or her feelings or deny the impact of the changes in the child's body and lifestyle. The child with learning differences may become the class clown to create diversion. Children may become so obsessed with thinness that they become isolated from social contacts and may have chronic body dysmorphism or confusion about their bodies that may last a lifetime. The chronic bed wetter may forgo sleepovers or camp and thus lose the social maturity of these experiences. The period is not latent but dynamic and active!

I recall so many families over my decades as a pediatrician and so many experiences with our own four sons and their friends. I have imagined this book as a guide for those whose lives are affected by children of this magical age. Frequently I encountered persons involved with children to be clueless about many of the common medical issues for this age range. I have aimed to gear the material for families, teachers, nurses, and therapists so that they may understand common illnesses and situations that may have crucial effects on the development of grade-school-age children. I hope that in sharing my knowledge, I have an effect on a child at this special time in his or her life.

CHAPTER 1

Fatima: A Ten-Year-Old Girl with Recurrent Headaches

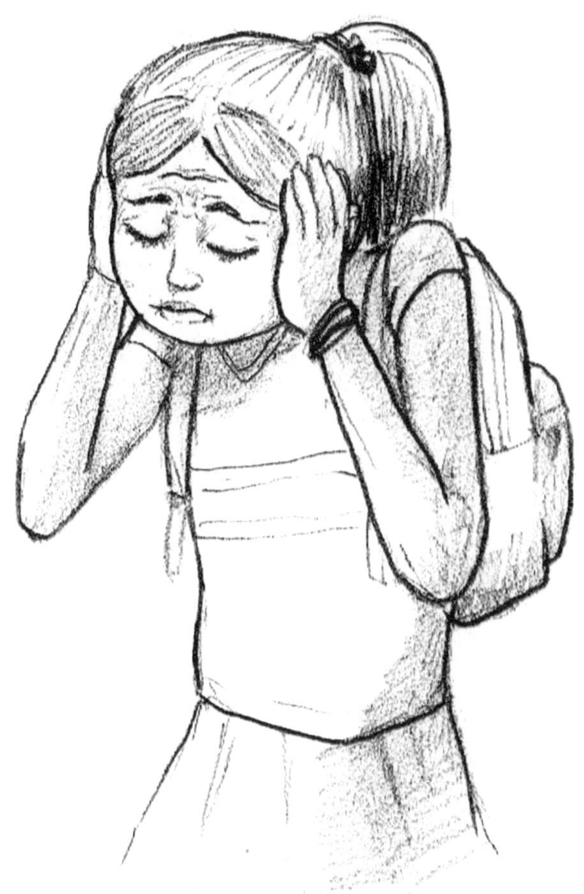

Fatima

FATIMA is a ten-year-old girl whose father calls me with a concern regarding her headaches. She recently told her father that her head pounds, and she feels like throwing up. She says she cannot go to school the next day. Similar episodes have occurred every few months for the last two years. Fatima's general health is excellent other than the headaches. She spent the night before her last headache at her friend's sleepover birthday party, and she recalls that she ate, "several pieces of pizza with pepperoni," and, "a lot of cake." The girls "stayed up very late" watching two movies on the computer monitor. Similar symptoms occurred on a prior sleepover and on several occasions over the last year. She feels like she cannot have any fun or go anywhere interesting because the activity might result in a headache.

I ask Fatima's father if there were recent unusual activities, if this headache differs from the previous episodes, if they have noticed any unusual body movements or behavior differences, or if any close relatives have recurrent headaches. Based on the history of no other symptoms and that the headaches are common in the family, I tell him that I think that this headache is probably in the migraine category. I reassure the father that migraines are usually treatable. I advise giving over-the-counter medication and making a doctor's appointment in the near future.

CLINIC VISIT

Fatima tells me she has taken ibuprofen and acetaminophen for the headache and has been able to fall asleep in a dark, quiet room. She is pain-free when she awakens in the morning. I ask more detailed questions about diet, sleep, medications, and health history, none of which is unusual. I give her a complete neurological exam. Although this exam is normal, Fatima's father is worried as his cousin's twelve-year-old daughter currently has a diagnosis of a brain tumor. He requests an X-ray or CT (computerized tomography) scan to be done as soon as possible.

Based on the above history and normal exam, I advise holding off on ordering an X-ray or CT scan. X-rays show skull bones but not bleeding or tumors in the brain. A CT scan shows many pictures of the interior brain, but it carries a significant risk of radiation. I also advise holding off on ordering an MRI (magnetic resonance imaging), which would probably require Fatima to have anesthesia to remain still during the test. I reassure the father that brain tumors are rare and that the symptoms of a tumor would be constant and increasing in severity.

I then discuss what the family should watch for when their daughter has another headache and what would necessitate imaging testing. I advise keeping a journal documenting diet, sleep, and anything unusual about the headache. I explain what triggers may be precipitating the headaches. I explain treatment options if over-the-counter medications are not effective. I tell him what changes to watch for and when to bring Fatima into the clinic.

HEADACHES IN CHILDREN

Headaches in grade-school-age children are fairly common. One percent of emergency room visits for grade-school-age children involve a headache.

Headaches may be categorized as follows:

- A primary headache, which means the symptoms are coming from the brain. Diagnoses are neurologically based, such as migraine, tension, mass lesions like a tumor or cyst, or cluster headaches.

- A secondary headache, which means something is acting from the outside of the brain. Causes are infections like viral upper-respiratory or sinus or ear infections; meningitis, which is an infection of the covering of the brain by virus or bacteria; bleeding from head trauma or from a weak vessel; or a tumor, which may be malignant (cancerous) or benign.

MIGRAINE

Migraine headaches affect 5 to 10 percent of grade-school-age children. Migraines are more common in boys until puberty, after which migraines are more common in girls.

Signs of a typical migraine headache are:

- Sudden onset
- One-sided location, although young children may have bilateral symptoms
- Recurrence
- Throbbing
- Hereditariness
- Strong need to sleep
- Cessation of symptoms with sleep
- Absence of other illness

Symptoms that sometimes occur prior to or during the migraine headache include:

- Nausea and vomiting
- Abdominal pain
- Flashes of lights or wavy lines
- Photophobia (discomfort to bright lights)

- Phonophobia (sensitivity to sound)
- Osmophobia (sensitivity to strong odors)
- Speech disturbance
- Dizziness or body imbalance
- Weakness of limbs
- Pale skin

Some children may have an aura preceding the above symptoms by up to sixty minutes. This prelude to the headaches is usually characterized by a flickering in the fields of vision or blurring of vision. The child may feel pins and needles on the face, numbness of one side of the face or body, decreased position sense, speech disturbance, or one-sided weakness. Although these signs may usually define a typical migraine, they may be very troubling to the family and create fears and anxiety of something happening that may be serious or life-threatening.

MIGRAINE CAUSES

The pathways from the above triggers to the actual pain receptors that pick up the signal are not yet fully understood. Researchers are currently studying the trigeminal nerve, located above and in front of the ear by the temples, and the trigeminal's neighboring nerves. A neuropeptide (protein) called CGRP (calcitonin gene-related peptide) is associated with this trigeminal nerve, which causes vasodilation (enlarging of the nearby blood vessels) and inflammation and the release of irritants, which is felt as pain.

Family members are often aware of the heredity component of the problem. Commonly a family member will recognize the symptoms but is surprised when the headache occurs in a child. The actual gene identification has only been found in the rare family with familial hemiplegic (paralysis on one side) migraine. As research advances, more specific gene identification is expected.

MIGRAINE TRIGGERS

- Excessive screen time, such as several consecutive hours on any electronic monitor of any size, such as a TV, pad, gaming box, computer, laptop, or smartphone
- Lack of sleep or change in the sleep environment
- Some food products, such as preservatives like nitrates found in packaged meats, or MSG, often used as a flavor enhancer
- Excessive sugar
- Travel to high altitudes
- Flashing or fluorescent lights
- Strong odors
- Menses in the pubertal girl
- Increased barometric pressure or weather changes
- Stress and anxiety, especially regarding auditions or testing

MIGRAINE TREATMENT

The treatment of migraine in children is both preventive before symptoms appear and emergent when pain is present. Learning about and avoiding triggers are the most important actions the family may take for the child.

Preventive medications are used when the migraine episodes are frequent and interfere with the child's social and school lives. Propranolol, a common treatment for hypertension, at a low dose is a commonly used daily medication. Anti-seizure medications or tricyclic antidepressants are occasionally used in difficult to treat cases. Botulism toxin or magnesium injected every few months along the trigeminal tract is helpful in adult migraines and may be a future treatment for children with migraines.

Emergent medications for a sudden onset of headache include the well-known over-the-counter medications ibuprofen (Motrin or Advil) and acetaminophen (Tylenol). Medications in the "triptan" (serotonin 5-HT 1B/1D agonist) group are frequently used in adults with migraines. Research outside of the United States shows effectiveness of the triptans if given early in the course of the migraine in children. Future research is expected.

Nondrug treatments of migraine in children have included acupuncture, biofeedback, stress management, and cognitive behavioral therapy. These modalities have not been researched for large groups of children.

I have learned that most children are able to feel better with over-the-counter drugs and cool compresses on the areas of the head affected and are able to fall asleep in a dark, quiet room. By far the majority of children with migraines are pain-free when awakened.

HEADACHE CAUSES OTHER THAN MIGRAINE

TENSION HEADACHES

Tension headaches are common in children. Statistics are not available as families rarely feel the need for the children to seek medical care. The child may describe the constant headache as feeling like a band being pulled across the face or forehead or pressure at the back of the head. They may describe triggers for tension headaches as a lack of usual sleep or of recent travel, school issues, or recent family stresses.

If a child has a tension headache, there will probably not be any of the migraine signs, such as nausea or vomiting, any signs of weakness or coordination problems, or sensitivity to light or sound. A neurological exam will not provide any worrisome findings.

Treatment for the child is rest, fluids, reassurance, and possibly an anti-inflammatory medicine, such as ibuprofen (Motrin or Advil).

CLUSTER HEADACHES

Cluster headaches are rare in grade-school-age children. The pain is severe and usually behind an eye. The symptoms may include nasal congestion, red eyes, swelling around the eyes, and unequal pupils. The pain may occur daily for weeks, lasting minutes or, rarely, hours. There may be pain-free months between episodes. Chronic pain without breaks in symptoms is the exception.

Treatment may include being injected with triptans (refer to "Migraine Treatment") or breathing 100 percent oxygen in the emergency department. Verapamil taken daily may be used as a preventive treatment.

INJURY TO THE BRAIN

A history of trauma followed by headache may result in:

- Nausea and vomiting
- Weakness on one side of the body
- Coordination problems
- Seizures
- Irritability
- Increased drowsiness
- Loss of consciousness
- No memory of the traumatic event

Any of the above symptoms are signs that child should be seen in an emergency department, and a CT scan will probably be ordered.

MALFORMATION OF THE VESSELS OF THE BRAIN

Bleeding can occur with or without trauma to the head if the blood vessels are tangled or if there is a weak area in the vessel wall (aneurysm). Symptoms may be severe headache; nausea and vomiting, especially in the morning; unusual behavior; and change in balance or movement. These abnormalities are rare.

BRAIN TUMORS

Of course this is every parent's fear when a child has a significant headache, especially if the child has some of the symptoms associated with migraine. As in Fatima's father's case, hearing about another child who has a tumor will exacerbate these fears as brain tumors are second only to leukemia and lymphoma in the age range of five to twelve years. Most parents have heard the frightening stories.

Brain tumors in children are usually found in the cerebellum, located at the back of the head. This area controls balance. The child may have an imbalance in muscle coordination. The child will probably complain of a headache and will be unusually irritable. The symptoms will steadily progress. Vomiting will likely occur in the morning and will be persistent.

Diagnosis will require a CT scan, an MRI, and possibly a biopsy of tissue. Treatment will vary depending on whether the cells are benign or cancerous and the tumor size and location. Over the past few years there have been important advances in precision of surgery, localized radiation, laser treatment, cryosurgery (freezing of the tumor), individualized chemotherapy, and immune therapy.

HEADACHES ASSOCIATED WITH INFECTIONS

Headaches frequently occur with common upper-respiratory viral infections. Fever may exacerbate the headache. In rare cases, the virus may migrate to the brain and cause encephalitis, an infection in the brain cells, or cause meningitis, an infection of the lining of the brain. The history of a cold sore or genital blisters in family members may lead to a diagnosis of herpes virus, which rarely causes an infection in the brain. Other common viruses—such as influenza, Zika, and West Nile virus—may occasionally infect the nervous system. An unvaccinated child may have a severe headache from the rubeola (measles) virus, varicella (chickenpox), influenza, or coronavirus (including COVID-19). The list of viruses that can cause neurological problems is extensive.

Bacterial infections may cause meningitis or abscesses in the brain. The most feared infection is meningococcal meningitis, which may be serious. Common bacteria like staph, strep, E. coli, and tuberculosis (TB) may cause neurological infections that lead to headaches. If the physicians feel a child may have meningitis, they will advise a spinal tap and possibly a CT scan to diagnose the infection and check for brain swelling.

Parasitic and amoebic infections that cause headaches are rare in children in the United States but may be considered if there is a history of travel or freshwater swimming.

THE DIFFICULT QUESTION: WHEN TO BRING THE CHILD INTO CLINIC

The family should bring the child in if there any of these symptoms:

- Persistent headache, nausea, or vomiting, especially after an injury
- Increase or change in the pain, especially if in the morning
- Unusual gait or balance problems
- Persistent change in behavior or personality without a known cause
- Confusion
- Frequent need for pain medication
- Fever with a stiff neck or with a severe headache
- A strong feeling that "Something is not right"

Diagnosis of the causes of childhood headache require a careful history of the child's symptoms and behaviors, a careful neurological examination by the provider, a CT scan, and possibly an MRI scan. Diagnosis is helped if the family keeps a journal of symptoms with descriptions, timing, and associated events.

FOLLOW-UP AFTER FATIMA'S OFFICE VISIT

Fatima's father understands that the triggers of migraine headache—such as lack of adequate sleep, too much junk food and electronic device watching—precipitate his child's migraine. Fatima and her family agree to watch for these situations and to treat the headache early with over-the-counter medications and adequate sleep. I suggest that Fatima and her father keep a headache diary, so they may be able to recognize more triggers for Fatima's headaches.

On the follow-up clinic visit, Fatima reports to me that she is able to decrease the frequency of her headaches by being careful not to spend hours on her iPad. Ibuprofen was helpful for her last mild headache.

Oh, to be pain-free.

RESOURCES FOR FAMILIES

- The http://americanmigrainefoundation.org is a site that has educational materials and support groups.
- Http://www.thedailymigraine.com/support-groups has Facebook connections.

CHAPTER 2

Maya: An Eleven-Year-Old Girl with Weight Loss and Social Isolation

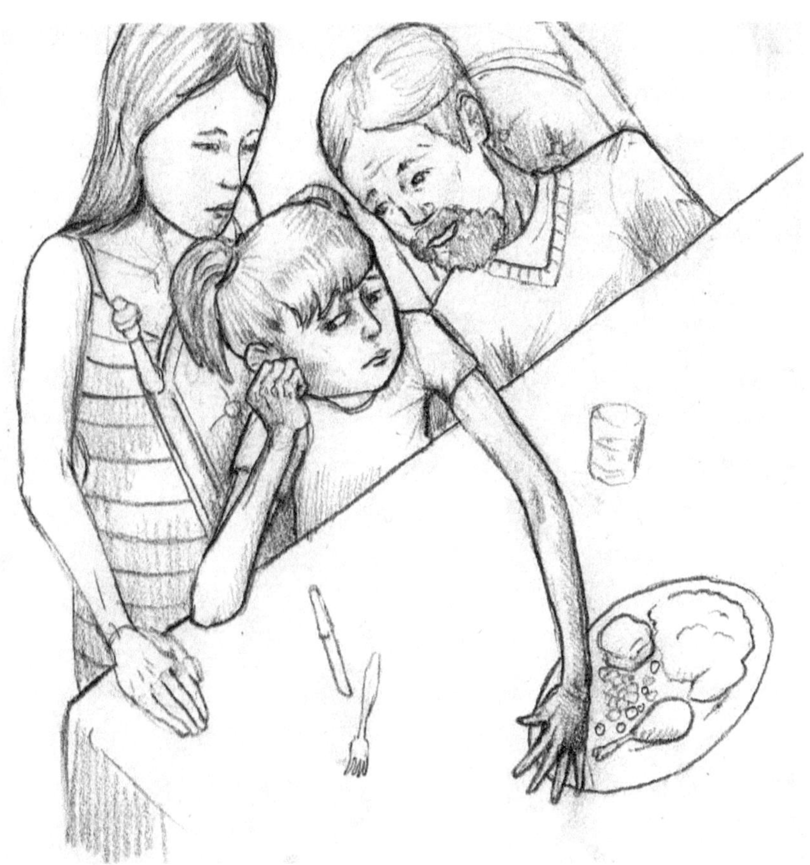

Maya

MAYA comes into our clinic with her family for her yearly physical. She needs a form completed for her ballet class that will confirm that she is in good health. Her father asks that they talk privately with me before the exam. He expresses concern that "Maya is obsessing about her weight and that she is too fat to be a ballerina. We feel she is too thin."

Her father says her only passion is the ballet. "We schedule our lives around Maya's dance lessons and performances. She has lost contact with her friends and no longer participates in any activities outside of the dancing. She says she wants to quit her demands at school because she does not need silly books to be a ballet star. Recently her ballet teachers are worried that Maya is not at a healthy weight for such strenuous dance exercise."

Maya's father describes his daughter as very hard working in everything she does, emphasizing that she is incredibly neat and tries for perfection in ballet. She recently stopped trying for the top grades in school. People often call Maya the "perfect child," but her father is worried because although Maya often talks about food, cooks for the family, and wants to do the grocery shopping, she is a very picky eater. He also says that Maya exercises until she drops from fatigue.

Maya's aunt was anorexic, and her grandmother has been diagnosed with obsessive compulsive disorder (OCD). Her mom feels that "Maya has become less social and often prefers to stay in her room. She has not wanted to have her friends over anymore. She becomes upset when I bring up the idea of calling or texting her old friends. She has not been invited to parties for a long time. Other mothers have begun to ask me if there is something wrong with Maya as she does not look or seems to feel well. I don't think she has an eating disorder. Something else is wrong."

THE CLINIC VISIT

When I ask Maya about any concerns, she says, "I am worried that my hips are too big, and my inner thighs are lumpy. Do you know any exercises to make my body thinner? I don't like being fat." However, she says that she does like food and loves to cook. When I ask her how much she eats, she becomes quiet and withdrawn.

I find in my exam that Maya's weight is in the third percentile, which means that 97 percent of children her age weigh more than she does. Her height is in the seventy-fifth percentile, which means that only 25 percent of children her age are taller than she is.

Her body mass index (BMI) is low for her age and her height, indicating that she is considered underweight. The BMI is calculated from a formula that uses a mathematical comparison of weight, height, and age. The BMI is then graphed on an age chart for further information about how the child compares to his or her peers. (Please refer to internet CDC BMI calculations.) When a child's BMI drops too low from healthy numbers, it is a cause for concern.

Maya's heart rate is fifty beats per minute, lower than expected for her age. Most children her age have a heart rate from eighty to one hundred beats per minute. However, some athletes have heart rates in the fifties. When a person's calories are too low for normal energy expenditure, the body tries to save energy and lowers the heart rate. For the same reason, the body temperature may be lower than expected. Fortunately Maya's temperature is normal. Her body is thin, and I can see the outline of her ribs. She has no signs of puberty. Her breasts, genitalia, and body hair are that of a younger girl.

Based on Maya's and her family's statements, her obvious thinness, and lack of signs of early puberty, I am worried that Maya has an eating disorder. I talk to Maya and her family about my concern of anorexia and my reticence to sign the ballet release papers. Maya becomes withdrawn, stares at the floor, and refuses to talk to me. Her father says that Maya often withdraws when the family tries to talk to her about the concerns of the ballet teachers and about her diet and exercise patterns.

EATING DISORDERS

I have learned that eating disorders occur in all socioeconomic and ethnic groups. Children with body image problems may be dangerously thin, have abnormal results of laboratory and heart tests, and may complain that they are too fat or swollen or bloated. They often occur in athletes, especially gymnasts and dancers, whose ideal is being thin. Children who have problems with body image have a disconnection about their body shapes or characteristics; this is also known as body dysmorphism. They are often in denial about the realities about their bodies. The most common eating disorders associated with weight loss are anorexia and bulimia.

Anorexia nervosa is an eating disorder in which the child has an error in body imaging, feels overweight, decreases normal eating, and actively tries to lose weight. The disorder is increasing in frequency and is occurring in children as young as five years old. As many as 1 in every 100 adolescents may be anorexic. Females are ten times more affected than males.

Anorexia nervosa is diagnosed when the following criteria are met:

- The child has an intense fear of becoming obese even when losing weight. She may have been previously obese and is overreacting to her new image.
- The child's perception of her or his body is very different from reality; that is, from how people see him or her.
- The child's weight drops by 15 percent as he or she gets taller without a medical reason for the change.
- A female child skips three consecutive periods, or a child from either gender has a delay of the onset of puberty.

Less-strict criteria for the diagnosis of anorexia are:

- Excessive exercise even when feeling weak
- Denial of hunger
- Preoccupation with food purchasing and preparation

My physical evaluation will often reveal extreme thinness and decreased muscle mass. Vital signs, like heart rate and blood pressure, may be low. Laboratory tests may show abnormal electrolyte levels, and tests may indicate anemia. When the body receives insufficient calories, fat and muscle cells are damaged, and levels of chemicals, like electrolytes—sodium, potassium, chloride, bicarbonate—are changed. Anemia will result if blood cells are not made in the usual number.

Some children may have excessive water intake to fool the family and the provider that they have gained weight. Rare causes of weight loss may be caused by cancer, thyroid issues, or other hormonal problems. This may result in abnormal lab values. These disorders will show signs other than those previously described. We will also check for other causes of weight loss before confirming the diagnosis of an eating disorder. Tests will be chosen based on history, clues, and physical examination of the child.

Bulimia is a disorder of body image in which the child

binges on food and then tries to lose weight by self-induced vomiting and purging with diarrhea. Bulimia is less common in children than in adolescents. Diagnosis is difficult as many children who binge and then self-vomit or use laxatives for rapid purging may maintain a normal weight.

Behaviors of bulimia that families may notice include:

- Leaving the table soon after a meal or after binging on snacks and then spending an unusual amount of time in the bathroom.
- Taking out his or her own garbage to hide evidence of binging or purging. Children may hide the chip or cookie bags. Children may use ipecac (used to treat poisoning by toddlers) to induce vomiting or may use laxatives for diarrhea. These are found in many families' medicine cabinets.
- Fixating on body weight or appearance.
- Having episodes of overeating or of fasting.
- "Pigging out" every day but not gaining weight.
- Thinning of dental enamel from acid erosion by vomiting stomach acid. Families or the dentist may notice a thinning, darkening, or easy chipping of the teeth. Dentists are often the first persons to consider bulimia in a child.
- Experiencing burning in the esophagus, the feeding tube between the mouth and the stomach. After vomiting, stomach acid will burn the esophagus, causing pain in the center of the chest and often malodorous breath.
- Having frequent bowel movements that may be caused by overuse of laxatives. The child may have diarrhea and then constipation.

Children and adolescents with either anorexia or bulimia often show signs of an obsessive compulsivity. They may be overly concerned about body image and cleanliness; have food obsessions, including color and texture; and have extreme exercise schedules. They may obsessively shop for food, cook for the family, and then eat little of the prepared food. The children may have an overwhelming interest in athletic activities, such as ballet or gymnastics, which have highly structured and formalized rules.

CAUSES OF EATING DISORDERS

The causes of eating disorders in children are complex. As in Maya's case, there are often genetic components. Her aunt was anorexic, and her grandmother had been diagnosed with OCD. Children who have been sexually or emotionally abused may try to ward off puberty by remaining thin. In most persons, the release of the hormones associated with puberty requires that a child be at a minimum weight. Children who do not weight enough may not show signs of puberty.

Emotional problems, such as anxiety or OCD, may result in an eating disorder. Using food as a means of control by eating less may give the child a feeling of having more leverage in a dysfunctional family. Children who have been obese and then lost weight may continue to deprive themselves of food. They may also have body image problems, such as body dysmorphism. Many children are affected by and wish to emulate the images in the media of ultra-thin actors and models.

Research scientists have studied neurological pathways in both obese and anorexic persons. MRI scans have been used to study the human brain of people with eating issues. In the brains of children with anorexia, there is a reduction of brain tissue, which is thought to be caused by damage from malnutrition. Some children with eating disorders have inadequate intake of calories, protein, carbohydrates, essential fats, vitamins, and minerals. They may be diagnosed with malnutrition.

Functional MRIs, which measure activity in the brain, have

shown that in children with anorexia who are presented with food, different brain areas are stimulated than in those without anorexia who were exposed to food. Children with anorexia have decreased blood flow in the temporal lobe of the brain, an area that is important for social interaction and mental health. They also have impaired visual and spatial abilities and impaired visual memory. These changes may exacerbate the child's abnormal sense of body shape and weight.

Changes in the brains of children with bulimia are similar to those of children with anorexia, but they are less pronounced. These brain changes are usually reversible after the child regains an adequate weight. Some children who retain these changes may have had these abnormalities prior to developing symptoms of anorexia. It is difficult to know which comes first—the bulimia or the brain changes.

Bulimia may be very difficult to diagnose. Children will usually deny the binging and purging behaviors, but if families are suspicious, they should look for evidence. This requires caution as trust is important in family relationships. Rarely is it wise to spy on children, such as looking in their wastebaskets, interrupting when they are using the bathroom for an extended period, and checking their social media and text pages. But in these cases, checking on the child may be appropriate. Anorexia and bulimia may be life-threatening conditions.

Unfortunately there are internet sites that promote and give hints about how to achieve extreme weight loss. Magazines, movies, and television often depict ultra-thin females as having the perfect shape. To counter these negative images, families may discuss and show photos of famous girls and women who have normal bodies, such as models in Spain who must have normal BMIs to work, college basketball stars who are fit and strong, or Olympic swimmers who are fit and muscular. Families may watch these athletes perform and note the beauty in full-figured persons. Recently, more large-sized dancers, actors, and comedians have been honored in reviews and award ceremonies.

TREATMENT OF EATING DISORDERS

Treatment of eating disorders can be difficult and needs to be individualized for each child. Clinics that specialize in children's eating disorders will ideally include a physician or nurse practitioner, a dietician, a psychotherapist, a specialized nurse, and a health educator. If the child has any underlying psychiatric problems, such as severe anxiety or depression, and may need medications, he or she will be referred to a psychiatrist.

My experience is that families are often in denial that their children are so ill. Everyone in the family needs to be in agreement about the plans made in a clinic session. Some families are very dysfunctional and often have conflict during mealtimes, which may counter any plans. Siblings may be jealous of the attention the affected child is now getting. Marital problems, alcohol or drug use in the family, excessive control behaviors, or physical, sexual, or emotional abuse may be factors that necessitate family therapy.

Some families are very proud of their child's success in activities such as ballet, gymnastics, or beauty contests. Thinness is usually prized in these fields. Fortunately, many coaches and instructors, such as Maya's ballet teacher, are aware of the need for healthy bodies and are changing the images of their athletes. However, many parents are fixated on the child's success and deny the health problems. The pressure on these children may be intense. The therapist is a crucial member of the team in these situations.

As part of the therapy, during the clinic sessions, we usually plan a "contract" with the child regarding intake of calories, decrease in intense exercise, increase of the heart rate, expectation of weight increase, and resumption of periods or the onset of menarche (starting her period) if she is in puberty. The contract might include the gain of a pound a week or increase of heart rate from forty to above sixty, and/or limiting exercise to thirty minutes every other day. In return for these successes, the child is allowed texting and phone or internet privileges.

The contract may also include changes for the family, such as only pleasant conversation at the dinner table. We advise no weighing at home, which might create conflict. Each contract must be unique to each family. If the child is improving in these areas, privileges are increased. The rewards may be increased electronics time, contact with friends, increasing exercise periods, or continuing the ballet lessons.

During weekly visits with the experts, the child's blood pressure and heart rate will be checked, and the child will be weighed wearing minimal clothing. I may suggest that the children urinate before being weighed as they may "water load" (drink excess water before the visit to add extras pounds). In some difficult cases, the child may need to be observed when urinating.

Blood tests may be necessary, If the child appears quite ill, I may order them to check for body chemicals like electrolytes, which may show cell damage if high or low, or anemia if the red blood cells are low. A blood test is usually done at the first visit to access the level of illness so that there may be a comparison if weight continues to be lost. If the child is steadily gaining, the lab tests may not need to be repeated.

A child may need to be hospitalized if the lab tests or heart tests are significantly abnormal. In these cases, the child's food intake and vital signs will be carefully monitored. A contract for follow-up clinic visits will be made, and educational and therapeutic sessions will begin.

A PLAN FOR MAYA

Maya's story and her physical exam are consistent with typical anorexia nervosa. Her father and grandmother agree that she needs a multidisciplinary approach in a specialized clinic. Unfortunately, her mother does not agree with them that Maya needs help. Another area of concern is the family history of eating disorders in relatives, which statistically increases Maya's risk for a severe eating disorder. Maya is young and intelligent and her illness is of fairly recent origin, which lowers her risk for severe disease. She is referred to a clinic that specializes in eating disorders.

FOLLOW-UP FOR MAYA

Unfortunately, Maya has a rough course and requires hospitalization when her weight and vital signs fall. In the hospital her calorie count and her cessation of exercise are carefully controlled. In this regimented setting, she is able to comply with her contract of eating a specified amount of food. Her weight increases, and she becomes more open with the therapeutic staff. She is able to have gradual electronic time with videos and a computer. She begins to ask to contact friends and to talk to other children who have sent cards.

Over time her mother learns about the complexities of anorexia and comes on board with Maya's plans. Hospitalization may be for weeks, until the child and family are able to understand the illness and especially to change how Maya views her body.

As eating disorders have a propensity to recur, her family and the professionals involved need to follow her closely for an extended time. Some children and families who have a smooth transition to health may need to be followed for about a year. Children with setbacks and a strong family history of eating disorders and chaotic families may need to be followed with a focus on eating disorders throughout childhood and adolescence. Although rare, hospitalizations may last months if the weight remains in a dangerous zone or there are many setbacks. Issues with insurance are complex and will not be addressed in this book.

Children with anorexia or bulimia are now recognized sooner than in the past due to media coverage, and as a result are treated earlier in the course of the illness. As the education for families about eating disorders is ideally very thorough during the initial crisis period, these families are aware to watch for the recurrence of symptoms. In an ideal world where the child heals and remains healthy, children and teens are seen yearly by a primary-care physician or nurse practitioner to ensure a state of continued health.

Thinness is not beauty!

Robustness is ideal!

RESOURCES FOR FAMILIES

- The National Eating Disorders Association (http://nationaleatingdisorders.org) is an organization that campaigns for treatment and funding. They provide information as needed and host informal events.
- The National Association of Anorexia and Associated Disorders (http://www.anad.org) is a nonprofit organization that gives treatment referrals and operates support groups, conferences, and events.
- The Academy for Eating Disorders (http://www.aedweb.org) is a global professional organization committed to research, education, and treatment of eating disorders and hosts professional conferences. Families might be interested in the new research.
- About Face (http://www.about-face.org) aims to empower girls and women to fight harmful media messages and body images.

CHAPTER 3

Aman: A Six-Year-Old Boy Who "Spaces Out" and Has School Problems

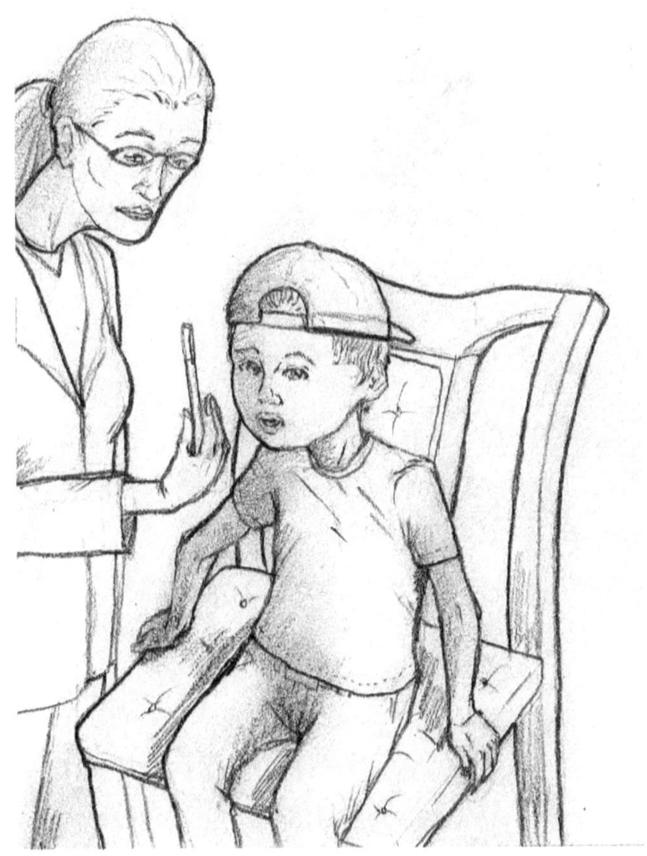

Aman

AMAN is a six-year-old boy whose mother is advised by his teacher that he is "spacing out" and has possible learning disabilities. Even in art period, he will leave a drawing half finished. The teacher advises that Aman see his medical provider. The teacher has written a note stating that she notices his learning curve is flattening as he often seems confused and cannot remember what has just been covered in class. At times he can read age-appropriate books, but he may just stare at the pages the next time a book is offered.

Aman's mother brings him to our clinic reluctantly saying he is just daydreaming. She feels he is very smart as he read at three years of age and loves his math homework. She says he does space out at times. She thinks it is just his active imagination that distracts him. These episodes began a year ago and now occur many times in a day. During these periods he just blankly stares off at an angle and does not focus for ten to twenty seconds. Sometimes his mouth will twitch a little or his eyelids flutter, but at other times, he just stares. He remains still and does not move or fall. He has no recall of what his mother says to him during these episodes. She feels Aman goes deeply into his daydreams. She has been reading about learning disabilities and feels that the label of "learning problems" does not fit Aman. She is worried that his teacher does not appreciate his curiosity and imagination or understand how bright he is. She is considering changing schools but feels his next teacher may also label him as "disabled."

Aman's mother says he has no health problems and has never been hospitalized. Aman eats and sleeps well and never seems unusually tired. He takes no medications, prescription or over the counter. He never has headaches or any problems with nerves or muscles. He has no behavior problems and has normal relations with his friends. He is as strong, flexible, and as coordinated as his friends. When asked about family history, his mother recalls his separated father once saying that he, "was a spacey kid." No one else in the family spaces out or has any neurological or psychological problems.

AMAN'S CLINIC VISIT

During the clinic visit, I assess Aman to be a healthy-appearing, friendly boy of normal height and weight. Questioning about his health does not reveal any health problems. I ask him about his "spacing out." He denies feeling any different before the spacing-out episodes. He is aware after the episode that something "felt wrong," but he does not remember what happens during the episode. "I am just gone." He says that sometimes he is teased about his daydreams, and his teacher seems upset with him. He does not remember, "doing anything wrong."

I complete Aman's physical exam with special emphasis on neurological testing. He appears completely normal except when I have him visually follow a moving pencil keeping his head still and using only his eyes. After some seconds as I move it back and forth, his eyes drift to the right and stop following the pencil movement. His eyelids flutter a little, his mouth drops open, and he seems unaware of his surroundings. His mother says this is the look Aman has when he is daydreaming. This event stops in about ten seconds. After a break, I try another diagnostic test. I ask him to breathe as fast as possible or pant like a dog. After a minute, the so-called spacing out repeats itself.

A little later I ask Aman if he will draw for me. I watch as he draws a simple figure of himself, his mother, dog, and house. He can print his name and talk about the picture. He reads a little in his book and willingly adds a few numbers for me. I inform Aman's mother that he is unlikely to have a learning disability but that he is missing important information during his events, and he must be very frustrated and confused in the classroom. I carefully explain that I think he may have a treatable seizure disorder, which can be confirmed by a painless EEG (electroencephalogram) test. A cap will be placed on his head to record his brain waves. I explain that he won't feel anything from the cap. I emphasize that this will probably resolve during his adolescent years, and his brain will not be damaged by the episodes. I tell the mother how smart I think he is and that I expect we will see a big difference for him in the future.

ABSENCE SEIZURES

Our brain's nerve cells communicate and signal by electrical charges. During a seizure (convulsion), the normal pattern of the signal changes to an abnormal pattern. A seizure can effect a small part of or the entire brain. If the entire brain is affected, the child will feel very tired after the seizure. But if the seizure lasts fewer than thirty seconds, the activity may not be noticed. The child may feel completely normal as the loss of consciousness is too short for awareness by the child.

Absence, previously called petit mal (little illness), is a brief seizure disorder that affects predominantly female children between the ages of three and eleven; it is rare in adults. The disorder occurs in 8 percent of children with epilepsy and second in occurrence to generalized or grand mal seizures. There are approximately 200,000 new cases a year in the United States. Unfortunately, these children have a 10 percent chance of developing another form of seizure disorder in the future.

This disorder is often missed as illustrated with my story of Aman. The child will completely blank out in episodes that may be rare or occur hundreds of times a day. The seizure will last twenty to thirty seconds and then stop abruptly. The episode is frequent during exercise. These children will stop moving but not fall. Their eyelids may flutter, their mouths may twitch or make chewing movements, and their hands make small movements, or rarely, make arm- and leg-jerking motions. The event passes quickly, usually in five to twenty seconds. The child will have no memory of the event.

Observers may think the child is purposely faking, daydreaming, or not paying attention. As the child is missing parts of surrounding communication and may be confused, he or she may be unable to learn school material. Children with this disorder may be treated as if they have a learning disability or a low ability to learn. Other children may not recognize that he or she may comprehend the visual and auditory signals in the environment and will be left out of group play. No brain damage occurs with this type of seizure, but the learning issues may be significant. The majority of children with absence seizures will react well with medications. Most children will outgrow this disorder in adolescence, with a resolution of their seizures in mid adolescence.

CAUSES OF ABSENCE SEIZURES

A third of children with this seizure type have a family history of absence seizures. Aman's father may have had absence, not just spaciness. Family history of absence is difficult to ascertain as the disorder is often missed, and the child usually outgrows the spaciness.

Other types of seizures may be short or only occur in one part of the brain. If the communication pathway of electrical signals in the brain is disrupted by malformation (change in structure) of the tissue, an injury, an infection, or a tumor, the electrical signals fire in an errant path, causing movement and behavior changes. Seizures may be focal, causing only one part of the body to behave abnormally, or grand, causing total body twitching and loss of consciousness.

The closest seizure to be confused with absence is a rare

temporal lobe seizure, which also may not be recognized by others. The temporal lobe regulates emotions and short-term memory. The child may seem to be awake and move around normally, or the child may pause as does Aman. The child with temporal lobe seizures may have personality changes, a headache, irritability, and an impending sense of doom. He will not remember the event. Careful history, observation, and EEG readings will differentiate these seizures. An EEG for absence will show abnormal general firing on both sides of the brain, not just in the temporal lobes.

DIAGNOSING ABSENCE SEIZURES

An EEG is the definitive test for absence seizures as there is a definite diagnostic pattern in these cases. The EEG detects the electrical signals in the brain and translates the signals to wave patterns that are diagnostic for absence. If there is any concern of other neurological problems, as with an abnormal exam, head injury, birth trauma, or brain infection, a CT, an MRI, or PET (positron emission tomography) scan may be preformed.

Some preteens or teens may be using street drugs that may mimic an absence event. A screen for these drugs may be warranted. Fortunately, Aman is only six years old!

Examination in the office will usually diagnose absence seizures with a high probability. The back-and-forth pencil movement and the rapid breathing tests, as done with Aman to trigger an event, are useful in a clinic setting prior to an appointment with a pediatric neurologist.

The underlying cause of absence seizures is unknown.

TREATMENT OF ABSENCE SEIZURES

Most children respond well to medications. Ethosuximide (Zarontin) or valproic acid (Depakote) are usually given with minimal side effects. Lamotrigene (Lamictal) may be tried as the above may have uncommon side effects such as dizziness, drowsiness, or intestinal symptoms. Families, friends, and teachers need to be educated about this disorder so that they do not judge the child to be a slow learner. Families, teachers, and health-care workers need to be aware of the symptoms of the absence disorder and guide Aman to understand he is not disabled.

FOLLOW-UP FOR AMAN

Aman's EEG shows the typical pattern for absence seizures. His MRI is normal without anatomic problems, masses, cysts, or any other abnormality. He is responding well to his medication and is showing a change in temperament. No longer does he seem confused or to be faking a lack of focus. His teacher is helping him to catch up with his academic work. His friends are beginning to include him in their activities. His mother was recently told by her sister that Aman's cousin had absence seizures, but the aunt did not understand the disorder and did not tell any friends or relatives. Fortunately, the cousin has grown out of the events.

It's always in the genes!

RESOURCES FOR FAMILIES

- Https://www.epilepsy.com/learn/childhood-absence-epilepsy is a site with excellent description of symptoms.
- Https://www.mayoclinic.org/diseases-conditions/epilepsy/symptoms-causes/syc-20350093 has information on causes, diagnosis, and treatment of absence.

CHAPTER 4

Adrian: A Seven-Year-Old Child with Wheezing and Disagreeing Divorced Parents

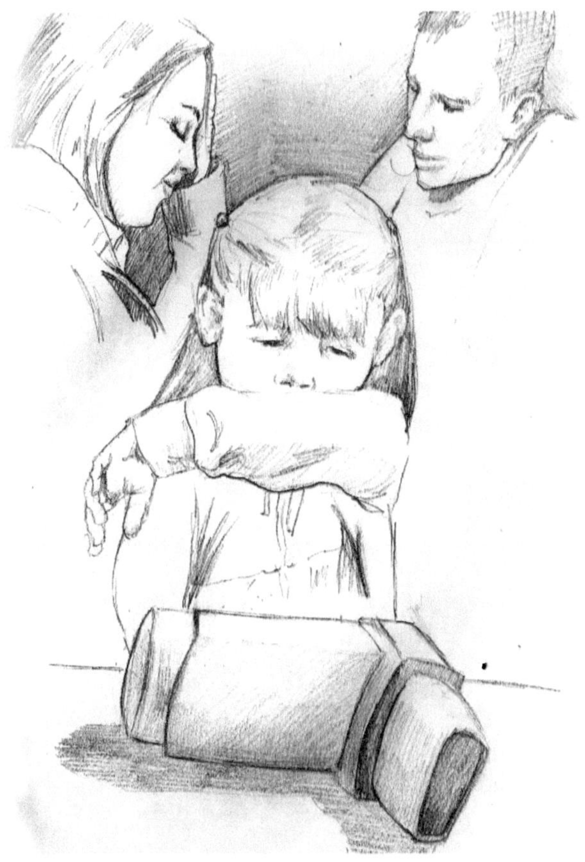

Adrian

ADRIAN is a young girl whose mother calls me as she is anxious about Adrian's coughing. "She coughs all the time and seems to be more tired than her friends." She brought Adrian to the emergency room a few days prior, at which time the doctor gave Adrian a medication to inhale. Adrian inhales the medicine as ordered for the next day and improves. Now she has spent two days with her father without using any inhaled medicine. Adrian's mother explains that she and Adrian's father are divorced, and they have shared custody. The mother is worried that her ex-husband has not followed through on giving the medication to Adrian and that she sleeps with two cats at Dad's house. Adrian's mother is calling me because Adrian's breathing seems labored, and she hears a whistling sound. I advise them to come to the clinic as soon as possible.

ADRIAN'S CLINIC VISIT

Adrian's mother describes her symptoms over the last day, while my medical assistant checks Adrian's breathing rate and heart rate, both of which are elevated as expected with her breathing difficulties. She then checks the oxygen level in her blood with a Band-Aid-like sensor on her finger. Her oxygen number is slightly lower than normal. Her blood pressure is normal. We then check her peak flow, a test of breathing into a tube that measures the amount of air being breathed out. Her flow number is lower than normal, indicating that her breathing tubes are constricted.

During these procedures, I listen to Adrian's breathing and hear equal sounding breathing with wheezing. I order a bronchodilator medicine to be inhaled. Within minutes, Adrian's breathing and her vital signs improve. Based on her story, vital signs, and symmetrical breathing, the diagnosis of asthma is confirmed. If I had heard unequal sounds, I would be concerned about an infection with fluid or an aspiration (breathing in something) of foreign material into one side of the lungs.

Adrian's physical exam other than her lungs is normal. Fortunately she improves after inhaling the medication. For some children there is a need for several inhaled treatments or for inhaled oxygen or a chest X-ray. Rarely will a child be hospitalized for continued evaluation and treatment.

Adrian's mother has done an internet search and agrees with me and the emergency room doctor that her daughter has asthma. She says that Adrian has always coughed more than her friends and has gotten out of breath sooner than her friends. She adds that sometimes when Adrian tries to run, her breathing makes a whistling sound. Her dad thinks she is fine and that she just needs to breathe more deeply when she is playing. He is planning on having her take yoga breathing classes. He denies that the cats cause her to wheeze.

OVERVIEW OF ASTHMA

Breathing is the way the body obtains oxygen and expels carbon dioxide. Oxygen is breathed in and is used in the body's biochemistry for cell growth and repair. Carbon dioxide is breathed out, a by-product of the body's biochemistry.

When someone breathes, several tube-like parts of the body, known as the respiratory system, are involved. These include the nose, mouth, and the large breathing tube called the trachea (windpipe). The trachea branches into smaller tubes called the bronchi. These bronchi branch off and become even smaller breathing tubes called the bronchioles. The bronchioles end at air sacs called alveoli. This is where oxygen and carbon dioxide are exchanged through very small blood vessels called capillaries. The carbon dioxide is then breathed out, and the oxygen is carried by the bloodstream to the cells. The heart is important as heart muscles provide the force and pressure to move the blood through the blood vessels to the cells.

The muscles around the neck and between the ribs also help pull air into the body and push out carbon dioxide. The nostrils may also open wider to allow more air to be inhaled. If the bronchi and the bronchioles are swollen, inflamed, and restricted, then less oxygen gets to the alveoli. This tightening of the bronchioles is often called bronchoconstriction or bronchospasm.

A child with an asthma attack will usually breathe with a wheezing and or whistling sound, often called an exacerbation or flare up. The whistling sound is made when air rushes through the tubes. This is similar to what happens when water flows through a hose. If water flows through a hose normally at full force, it makes a certain sound. If the hose is squeezed and the water cannot flow through as easily, it makes a different sound.

When the child's breathing tubes, the bronchi and bronchioles, tighten or constrict, the child has to breathe faster than usual to get the amount of oxygen the body needs. The muscles between the ribs work harder and faster. The extra work being done by these muscles can be seen as these muscles between the ribs are sucked in. This sucking in is known as retraction.

Occasionally a child may just seem short of breath. This means the child will be breathing more rapidly than usual. The child will appear to be working harder to get air as the chest moves more forcefully, and retractions may be seen.

The child may just cough. Coughing is the body's way of attempting having to force open the bronchi and bronchiole breathing tubes. If the constriction is very severe, the child may not make a wheezing sound because there is so little air flowing through the tubes. Because asthma is not painful and the wheezing may not be heard, the family needs to watch for other signs, such as tiredness and shortness of breath.

Families may notice that their child's heart beats quickly during an asthma attack. A fast heart rate indicates that the lungs are working harder to bring more oxygen. The heart is pumping more to bring that oxygen faster to the cells of the body. The child's blood pressure may also be affected. A child with low blood pressure is very ill and needs to be seen in an emergency room. The child will be very quiet, appear tired and pale, irritable, and breathing with difficulty. During an asthma attack, a child may appear pale because the blood is carrying less oxygen.

Families may be surprised that the child seems ill but has no fever. Fever is a protective way for the body to keep bacterial or viral infections at bay. Occasionally there will be an infection and possible pneumonia associated with the asthma disease. The provider may hear the signs of an infection with a stethoscope and may choose to order an X-ray.

CAUSES OF ASTHMA

Asthma is triggered by environmental factors, irritants like allergens from nuts and seafood, and infections, especially viruses that cause the common cold. These triggers cause the immune system cells in the respiratory system to release irritating chemicals that cause swelling and mucous production in an attempt to rid the body of the triggers. Environmental irritants may also cause asthma. Smoke from cigarettes, fireplaces, woodstoves, and perfumes may cause increased visits to emergency rooms during "Spare the Air" days. Tobacco smoke, in particular, may linger on hair or clothing and persist as an irritant. Dust from garages, closets, thick carpeting, draperies, and feather pillows and mattresses may trigger asthma.

Allergens are a common cause of asthma. Allergens are triggers like animal hairs, pollution, dust, plant pollen, or some foods which may cause an allergic reaction in a child. These reactions may be sneezing or itching but may cause wheezing. Dander shed from cats, dogs, horses, and rabbits is a common trigger for wheezing. Some children are sensitive to mold, which may be found in damp areas of the home. When the source of the reactions is unclear, the child may need skin and/or blood testing in an allergy department.

Other causes of asthma may be sudden changes affecting the lungs, such as exercising, laughing hard, crying, or rapid changes in temperature. These changes act as mechanical triggers in the bronchi, causing them to tighten. Because crying and laughing may set off the constriction, families sometimes think that asthma is caused by emotion or stress. However, the effect is actually mechanical, not psychological. Stress does not cause asthma. There are also genetic factors at play for a child with asthma.

In the last century, asthma was considered to be reversible, but research over the last few decades has shown that untreated constriction and inflammation of the bronchi and bronchioles may lead to chronic lung disease.

I have found that families are often worried that something other than asthma is causing the symptoms. Wheezing does not always mean asthma. Uncommon causes of wheezing are some forms of heart disease, infection, or inhalation of something into the lungs. These can be identified by other symptoms, history of the child's health, physical examination, and imaging such as CT scans.

TREATING CHILDHOOD ASTHMA

I know that it is important for a family to learn how to tell if their child with asthma needs urgent treatment. Therefore I will individualize an asthma care plan that describes symptoms to watch for and actions to take. Signs to look for include wheezing and coughing, rapid breathing, paleness, irritability, tiredness, or retraction of the rib muscles. If the child is able to use a peak flow meter, a range of numbers will be on the plan.

The asthma care plan needs to be individualized for each child. Download a sample plan from the CDC website, <https://www.cdc.gov/asthma/actionplan.html>, or just look up "asthma care plan." The plan is usually divided into three zones: Good Zone as the child is well with no symptoms and can continue on none or on daily medications; Caution Zone means mild symptoms are present and controlling meds should be started; Danger Zone means symptoms are severe, and the child needs to increase medications and go to the emergency room or clinic.

Some children have a sudden wheezing reaction to exercise or to an allergen. These children can be treated with a "rescue" medication that they inhale, such as albuterol, which relaxes the bronchial tube muscle. Because albuterol helps open the airways, it is known as a bronchodilator. The rescue inhaler may need to be used only once, but some children use it for days or weeks as needed.

Some children may need to use an inhaled bronchodilator before exercising. They may use albuterol; or they may use cromolyn, which stabilizes the inflammatory cells. Other children may need to use this medication for a few years every time they play sports, while others may need it only when they have an upper-airway respiratory infection and wish to exercise. Most teachers and coaches are aware of the signs of asthma and when to give the medication to the child. If necessary, an inhaler and a note from the child's doctor with instructions can be kept at the child's school.

A child with an infection who is exposed to a trigger for a long time or who has frequent flare-ups may need to use a "preventive" inhaled corticosteroid for days or weeks to keep open the bronchi. These steroids are not the type featured in the news for muscle development. Since they are inhaled, only a small portion enters the bloodstream, thus they do not cause typical steroid side effects. Commonly used inhaled corticosteroids are budesonide, fluticasone, beclomethasone.

I may also consider prescribing a combination inhaled drug with one of these corticosteroids and a long-acting bronchodilator such as Salmeterol. Some children may be prescribed an oral drug such as montelukast, which acts by blocking a substance called leukotriene that causes bronchial inflammation. These medications cannot stop a sudden flare-up of wheezing. They are used to prevent attacks and for long-term control.

Some children need to use rescue medications only a few times a year and never need the preventive medications. Others may need daily preventive medications. Rarely, a child may need to use preventive medications for a few years. Each child needs an individualized treatment plan so that the medications can be tailored to match the symptoms.

The best way to get the most from these inhaled medications is with a spacer device. Most children cannot coordinate their breathing with the inhaler alone. With the spacer device the child is able to breathe the medication into a small plastic chamber that holds it so that the child may continue to breathe it in. The particles of medication are then inhaled more evenly into the lungs. This ensures the child gets the correct dose.

If the child's allergies cause significant problems, allergy shots, immunotherapy injections, may be needed. If this is the case, I may refer the child to an allergy clinic.

As part of a child's treatment, the family may receive printed material, watch a video about asthma, take an asthma class—where the child and family learn about the signs of asthma and the use of the inhaler and spacer—and be given an individualized care plan that specifies the signs and symptoms to watch for, especially if the child needs to avoid triggers, change medications, or come to the clinic.

SUMMARY OF ASTHMA MEDICATIONS

PREVENTIVE MEDICATIONS

- Inhaled *corticosteroids* include beclomethasone, budesonide, fluticasone. Side effects are rare. There is a possibility of an oral yeast infection in the mouth. Rinsing the mouth after inhalation of this will prevent the yeast.
- Oral *leukotriene receptor antagonists* include montelukast. This oral medication works by stabilizing irritated immune cells and are used to prevent bronchial inflammation when the usual regimen of inhaled corticosteroids and inhaled bronchodilators is not helpful. Side effects are rare.
- Inhaled *long-acting bronchodilators* include salmeterol and formoterol. These must be used only once a day. More frequent use can cause a dangerously rapid heart rate.

RESCUE MEDICATIONS:

- Inhaled *short-acting bronchodilators* include albuterol. This medication is known as a beta agonist and works by opening or dilating the muscles of the bronchi and bronchioles. Reversible side effects include an increased heart rate and mild tremor. These side effects are lessened with the more expensive levalbuterol.

- Other inhaled *bronchodilators* include ipratropium which is often used in a clinic or Emergency Room in conjunction with albuterol. Side effects include reversible increased heart rate and tremor.

MEDICATIONS FOR SERIOUS FLARE-UPS

Oral or injected *corticosteroids* include prednisone and dexamethasone. These may be given in a physician's office or an emergency room. An asthma care plan should state when the child might need them. Long-term side effects are unlikely to occur when these medications are only used to treat exacerbations. Reversible side effects of these corticosteroids may include irritability, a change in sleeping patterns, and increased appetite.

OTHER TREATMENT OPTIONS

Many families are opposed to the use of Western pharmaceutical products and wish to use "natural" treatments. Alternative or nontraditional medications are used by 80 percent of US families for minor symptoms and as a complement to treatments for major illnesses. Universities and educational conferences are adding courses in herbal and holistic medicine and other alternative approaches.

Parents are often frustrated by the chronic and recurrent nature of asthma. Because asthma is so common, parents hear about alternative treatments from friends or read about them online or in magazines. The negative press about some drug companies often causes parents to reevaluate their children's treatment plans and add alternative modalities.

Although breathing exercises, herbs, homeopathic medications, and acupuncture have been used to treat many childhood illnesses, a serious asthma flare-up is life-threatening, and modern science is lifesaving.

Alternative medications have side effects, just as do Western medications. Care must be taken when using these treatments, and all of them must be evaluated carefully by families who give them to their children. Signs of a severe asthma flare-up must never be ignored as children may die from respiratory failure.

Acupuncture has not been shown to have health benefits for treating asthma.

Biofeedback has been shown to decrease the occasional panic associated with an asthma flare-up.

Breathing exercises and *yoga* have anecdotally been reported to have been helpful in adults with asthma, but anecdotal reports are the weakest form of evidence.

Coffee and *tea* contain caffeine, which acts as a mild anti-inflammatory (anti-swelling) agent. Using coffee or tea in very young children is obviously not appropriate. Adolescents have found caffeine to be helpful.

Herbs such as ding-chuan tang, ginko, and lobelia are used in Chinese medicine to decrease wheezing and are considered by some providers as a treatment for mild symptoms. Ma huang, also known as ephedra, is banned by the US Food and Drug Administration (FDA) and should be avoided. There has been little research on herbal medications as they are considered foods, not medications, by the FDA.

Vitamin C and *vitamin E* act as anti-inflammatory agents and possibly have some effect in treating asthma. However, so far there is no evidence of their effectiveness.

ADRIAN'S FOLLOW-UP

Adrian's mother agrees to make sure that Adrian uses the medications and plans for them to attend an asthma class. As expected, Adrian's father is hesitant at first, but after he learns that asthma could be life-threatening, he agrees that it is worth trying the medications. He has also read about asthma and concurs that she might be sensitive to the cats. Adrian responds well to treatment with inhaled albuterol until she stops wheezing and two weeks of inhaled steroids to stop the inflammation. She resumes soccer with enthusiasm. She learns how to use a peak flow meter. Her father learns more about the treatments from the internet and videos. Both parents agree to watch Adrian carefully and to encourage her to use inhaled medications as needed. After her lung inflammation decreases over a two-week period, her asthma episodes become rare. The cats have a new loving home. Adrian decides that she will be a doctor when she grows up. "I will fix kids so they can breathe!"

I bet she succeeds!

RESOURCES FOR PARENTS

- The Allergy & Asthma Network Mothers of Asthmatics (www.allergyasthmanetwork.org) is a thirty-year-old nonprofit organization providing outreach, education, and research.
- The Asthma and Allergy Foundation of America V (www.aafa.org) is an over one hundred-year-old organization that provides education, support groups, research, and advocacy.
- The National Institute of Allergy and Infectious Disease (www.niaid.nih.gov) is a US government agency that provides major support for scientific research.

CHAPTER 5

Jaime: An Eight-Year-Old Boy with School Behavior Problems and Possible ADD

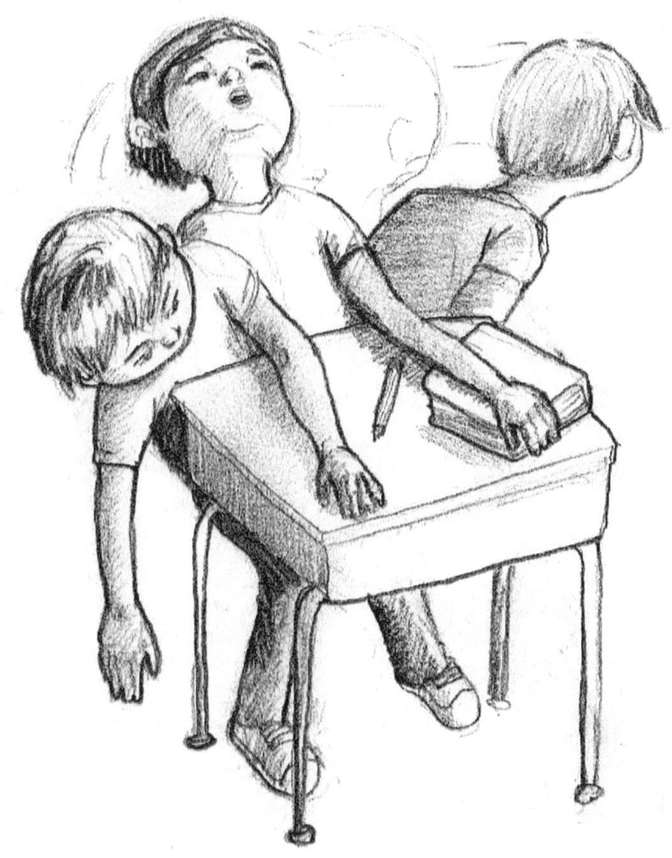

Jaime

JAIME is brought into my clinic by his mother who says that he may, "have to change schools again." At a recent parent-teacher conference, his teacher and a clinical school psychologist describe Jaime's behaviors. They say that Jaime taps his pencil and his feet many times an hour and shakes his head frequently. He sometimes makes odd humming noises. He keeps asking the other students for the assignments. These actions bother the other students and are unacceptable in the classroom. His academic progress in school is faltering. Jaime may need to repeat second grade.

The psychologist suggests that the school do an IEP (individualized educational plan) for him to test and assess for learning disabilities. His mother states that she has concerns that he will be labeled as "different" or "retarded" if he is tested. She knows he is active and has poor attention span. However, she feels he is smart and just needs to learn to focus. He has no trouble with his math homework because it seems like a fun puzzle to him. His weak areas are reading and writing, which easily frustrate him.

Jaime becomes fixated and hyperfocused while playing a video game in which he creates villages and cities with unique cultures. He adds exceptional buildings to the game environment and creates unusual humans and animals who live in his fictional world. He is able to play the game for hours and has advanced beyond his older siblings' gaming skills. He almost seems to be in a trance state when he plays, and he may become upset when he is pulled away from the game.

He has problems planning his homework and organizing his backpack and possessions. He often has his homework in his pack but forget to hand it in at school. He may lose his papers or books while searching for something else. He may become frustrated and tear up papers, which escalates the situation.

Jaime always seems to be more active than his siblings. He sleeps more fitfully, is more particular about food, and is more sensitive to temperature changes and to the texture of clothing. He seems to be less coordinated than his siblings in group sports. Her has more success with solo sports, such as bike riding and swimming.

Jaime has few friends. His mother thinks this may be because he does not catch the clues of group play. He interacts best with younger children as he can initiate and plan the activities. His problems with friends occur when he is impulsive or becomes upset if rules or sports or game activities are changed. His mother has noticed that he prefers time with an adult as he can focus better with a one-on-one situation and that adults may be more patient than his peers.

The recent separation of his parents has increased his active movement and poor sleep patterns. Jaime and his brothers are deciding now which parent's house they prefer. His mom says the stress of the household changes is negatively affecting Jamie's behavior. His self-esteem seems to be decreasing, and he often refers to himself as "stupid".

JAIME'S CLINIC VISIT

Jaime interacts well with me and asks lots of questions about the stethoscope and blood pressure cuff. He talks a bit about school and that he knows he is bothering his classmates. "I cannot stop. I try." When I ask what his favorite thing to do for fun, he answers that he loves his video game and proceeds to talk excitably about his detailed game world.

I assess that Jaime is a healthy and curious boy. He moves around the exam room, touching furniture and objects, with more movement than does the average eight-year-old. Jamie's exam is completely normal, with special emphasis on the neurological exam. Vision and hearing are normal. Deficits in these areas sometimes cause a child with attention difficulties to miss instructions and become frustrated.

In cases like Jaime's, I pay special attention to my evaluation of his fine motor function, his balance, and his symmetry of movement. I explain to his mother that we need to be sure that he does not have any underlying abnormality in his brain that would require an MRI.

ATTENTION DEFICIT DISORDER

Attention deficit disorder (ADD) is a neurological brain disorder in which there is a deficiency of the neurotransmitters norepinephrine and its precursor, dopamine. ADD affects approximately 6 percent of children between the ages of five and twelve. This disorder is characterized by the following:

- Lack of focus. The child may not be able to work on a task longer than a few moments and then will squirm and fidget. Even with breaks in the work, he or she may not be able to finish a section of homework. Children with ADD may have one or two areas in which they are able to work for hours, such as building a structure or playing a specific video game. But they are easily distracted and lack patience for projects.
- Lack of organization. He or she may not focus on instructions so homework may be late or disorganized. The child will lose papers and assignments, or take them to school but forget to hand them in. He or she will often lose articles of clothing, toys, and papers.
- Ease of distraction. The child may be very sensitive to noises. Even the sound of a car starting or a door closing will cause him or her to lose focus. Some children

with ADD find that steady background music is helpful; others find it too distracting.

- Repetitive actions. In an attempt to stay on focus the child may do annoying repetitive actions such as tapping, humming, blinking, or head bobbing. The child's gait or running style may seem awkward compared to others in his or her age group.
- Impulsive behaviors. The child may interrupt his teachers or classmates without awareness of the effect on them. He or she may engage in risky behaviors. Children with ADD may be unaware of the consequences of their body actions on bicycles or in pools.
- Overreaction to stimuli. Children may be very bothered by uncomfortable clothing, lack of sleep, hunger, or temperature changes. As infants they may have been difficult to soothe, to help fall asleep, or to tolerate a change of diet.

ADD/ADHD TYPES

- ADHD (H = hyperactivity) may be diagnosed by the above with the addition of activity that is extreme for the setting. The hyperactivity may be repetitive or sudden and unpredictable.
- ADHD may include impulsivity. The child may be unable to control certain behaviors, stop sudden actions, or interrupt others. He or she may blurt out words or answers in class.
- ADD defines the inattentive type, which has the above without the hyperactivity component. This form is more common in females. It may be difficult to diagnose as the child is often quiet and tries to cover for the lapses of focus. This form of ADD may be considered if testing eliminates learning disabilities as the cause for the

child's ease of distraction, lack of focus, and organizational problems.

MYTHS ABOUT ADD/ADHD

The myths about ADD result in late diagnosis and lack of help for these children. The child is often labeled as lazy or as lacking intelligence. ADD is a real biological disorder, not caused by poor parenting or family dysfunction. A child with ADD may have high intelligence, especially in one area, such as the creative arts. ADD does occur in girls. The child may outgrow the symptoms of ADD, but it may persist throughout life. Some with ADD are not diagnosed until they are in their thirties!

CAUSES OF ADD/ADHD

The risk of ADD in a child is increased if the child was born prematurely or exposed before birth to nicotine, alcohol, or street drugs. Early childhood exposure to high levels of lead or other toxins may cause symptoms of ADD. By far the highest risk factor is genetic. Usually a parent, sibling, aunt/uncle, or cousin has a history of lack of focus and lack of organization with resultant school problems. A relative may have frequent risky behaviors or impulsive actions. Often these relatives are never formally diagnosed.

CONFUSION OF ADD/ADHD WITH AUTISM

ADD crosses over with learning disabilities and some aspects of autism. Children with learning issues, like dyslexia, often lack focus and become distracted easily from their tasks because of the energy it takes to finish the reading.

Autism is a disorder with issues of poor verbal communication and social skills. These children have many characteristics, mainly poor eye contact, delayed speech, and problems with nonverbal cues. They overlap with ADD in strong reactions to stimuli and risk-taking behaviors during play. Diagnosis using an IEP and psychological evaluation will determine if the ADD child has some learning disabilities and/or autism characteristics.

DIAGNOSIS AND TREATMENT OF ADD/ADHD

The diagnosis of attention problems is made by trained pediatricians, nurse practitioners, psychologists, psychiatrists, and MSW social workers, all of which require special training. These professionals may use the Continuous Performance Test, the Connor's Check List, an IEP, and/or the SNAP rating scale. Genetic history, teacher information, a neurological exam, an IEP, and psych evaluation usually define the diagnosis of ADD. Treatment of ADD is mainly based on increasing focus and organization.

Having fixed daily routines and creating a safe and quiet environment for study are primary. Decreasing TV and gaming use, even considering having these available only on weekends, is often beneficial. Using gaming time as a reward for successes might be helpful for Jaime. The child with ADD needs a quiet space and scheduled breaks with the use of a timer. Advance warnings of schedule changes are important. Sticky notes with reminders on his backpack, paper files for his backpack, having a space near the door for his finished work (and his lost shoes) may also be helpful. A checklist for his activities and assignments may help make sure necessary things are accomplished. Attempting to increase organization at home may be helpful for everyone, including siblings.

Discussion with Jaime's teacher about breaking assignments

into smaller pieces, having him sit closer to the front alongside quiet children and showing him how to organize his desk with a few paper folders may be helpful. Written assignments rather than oral ones may help Jaime organize his work. Frequent meetings with the teacher and experts in the field to assess if changes are helping are important. Most children are reassured that they are now understood and that they are not "stupid". Knowing that ADD is a real diagnosis with treatment options helps the child to feel more confident.

Social skills are difficult for the child with ADD to learn. Impulsivity, emotions on the edge, and problems with transitions create problems. Having an activity planned for a playdate may be helpful in providing structure. Keeping a schedule for social activities may aid the child with ADD to maintain focus.

MEDICATIONS FOR ADD/ADHD

The question of medications for ADD always comes up, usually from discussions with the teacher who has seen many children become much calmer on the drugs. Parents are often worried that their children may become addicted, and they prefer to wait for them to outgrow their behaviors. In my experience, I have only observed calmness in the child without signs of addiction. Age of the child and the extent of school and social problems should determine the use of drugs. Families need to know that children may only need a few months or a year on the medications to attain more focus and organization.

Each child with ADD is unique, and each may have a different reaction to the medications. Going slowly with doses and patience is important. The most common forms of ADD/ADHD medications are amphetamines and methyphenidates. There are many brand names for drugs that contain either of these. They may be in liquid, tablet, or capsule form. They may be short acting, extended release, or long acting. Some children take a long-acting medication before school and a short-acting one for homework time. Some children need a midday medication given by a school nurse. Some families forgo medications on weekends and holidays. If the above amphetamine or methylphenidate medications have side effects such as increased heart rate, lack of appetite, or sleep disturbances that persist after a few weeks, nonstimulants such as atomoxetine or clonidine medications may be tried.

Side effects are frequent for the first few days or weeks of treatment, so patience is required to evaluate whether to change medications or modify dosage of a drug. Headaches or nausea my occur but will usually lessen after few days. Tics, unusual mouth or body twitchy muscle movements, usually require changing the medication. The child may have mood changes or become too sedated and may need change in dose or med to dissipate. Sleep issues are common and may result in needing to give the short-acting medication earlier or try the extended-release form in the morning. Many children who take the extended-release med in the morning may not be hungry for lunch. Either breakfast needs to be larger, or the medication may be changed to short release early and short acting in the afternoon.

Many parents are fearful for their hyperactive children to take a stimulant drug. It seems counterintuitive for this to work, but these medications stimulate the neurotransmitters to increase, and the neuron communication calms the hyperactivity.

FOLLOW-UP ON JAIME

Jaime's parents are currently separated, but both agree that they need to help Jaime during this time. They have agreed on custody issues. The plan is to have housing near each other with the boys splitting their time on a structured schedule. They are trying to help with organization and work with Jaime on breaking up tasks and assignments for a while. If there is no improvement by middle school, they have agreed to try the medications. They have scheduled a therapist to help him with the separation, school problems, and his self-esteem.

Jaime seems to be doing better with lots of structure at his homes and a cooperative teacher, who has moved his seat location and has helped him with his backpack organization. A few recent playdates in the park with lots of running around and playing on structures have been successful.

All kids lose their homework. And their shoes!

RESOURCES FOR PARENTS

- Https://www.healthychildren.org/English/health-issues/conditions/adhd has good information and resources.
- Https://childmind.org/guide/what-parents-should-know-about-adhd has a good discussion of the diagnosis and treatment of ADD.

CHAPTER 6

Halley: A Twelve-Year-Old Girl with Tiredness and Obesity Issues

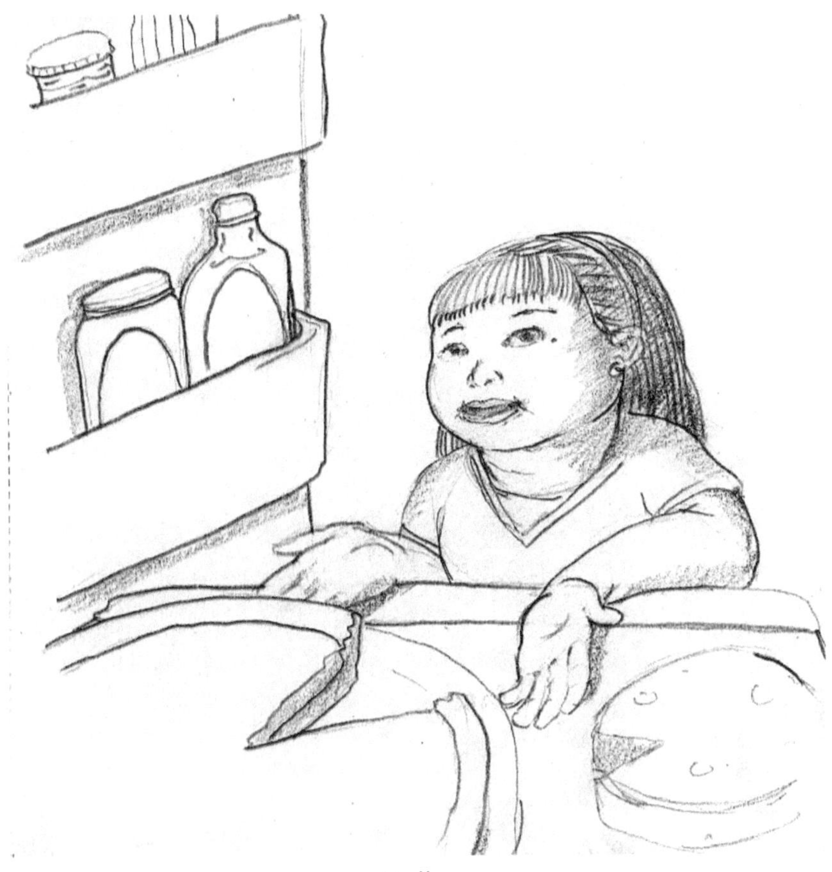

Halley

HALLEY and her mother come to see me with concerns about Halley being too tired to do her usual activities or her homework. I ask Halley and her mother questions about recent and past illnesses, sleeping patterns, her level of exercise, and any symptoms other than being tired. I notice she is overweight for her age. I ask about her weight, but Halley is reticent to talk and starts crying. After a few minutes she begins to talk. "They tease me in gym class. Being fat is dopey and stupid." She talks about feeling guilty every time she eats junk food but cannot ignore the urge to eat the food. Sometimes she cries when she sees all the skinny girls in magazines and on TV. She feels left out of sports because she cannot keep up with the other kids and is always last to get picked. She is too tired to finish her homework, so she is falling behind in class. She feels like she does not have any friends and dreads going to school.

Halley's mother explains that her daughter was just a little pudgy until puberty, when she started to gain weight. She says she is not worried about her daughter's weight, just her tiredness. "We are all big people. She was born big." Her mother feels that food is a comfort to Halley and that she is calmer after eating pizza or ice cream. Halley's sister has just left home for university, and Halley cries about missing her and then binges on food.

The mother recalls that an aunt has low thyroid, and several cousins who are large have diabetes. She says that everyone in the family is large and healthy: "My own diabetes test (HgA1C) is high, but I feel great." She feels that Halley needs a test for hormones but does not want her on a diet. She has known several girls who lost a lot of weight and then become too skinny.

THE CLINIC VISIT

I carefully note Halley's height and weight and compare the numbers with her prior measurements and those of other girls on a comparison chart. Her height is increasing at a normal rate, but her weight is increasing at a faster weight than that of her age peers. Her heart rate is normal. Her blood pressure is slightly higher than the normal blood pressure for her age.

Halley's physical is normal other than her obesity, her elevated blood pressure, and some darkening of the skin on her neck. Her breasts and body hair are consistent with a mid-puberty stage. She seems sad and is tearful. She appears not to feel okay about her mother's denial of the overweight issue. I suggest that she might be interested in talking in a group with some other children her age who are having trouble at school with teasing. I describe a program we have in clinic that includes a nutritionist, a health educator, and a therapist to help her feel stronger, less unhappy, and less tired. She asks her mom if she may go to the group. "I gotta lose weight."

OVERVIEW OF OBESITY

Social and cultural issues are always present regarding body size. In the deep past, heavy women were prized as they represented the wealth of a family. In primitive cultures, a few women were grossly overfed to illustrate the wealth of the chief of the tribe. From the Stone Age to the early 1900s, obesity was viewed as a sign of beauty and prosperity. The art of the Renaissance period illustrates the status of the overweight female. Now that the ultra-thin model and actress are revered, there is significant discrimination against the obese. I am careful in the clinic to cover issues of obesity with tactful evaluation.

I have observed that obesity in children has become a major issue in health care in the last thirty years. Obesity is defined as a BMI (basal metabolic index) at or above the 95th percentile for age and 85th–95th percentile as overweight for age. There has been a 30 percent increase in overweight children and adolescents in the last thirty years. There are estimates that in the United States, one in twelve preschoolers and one in six grade-school-age children are obese. Obesity affects not only physical health but also social and emotional states, leading to depression and low self-esteem.

Factors causing this epidemic may be simplified to a child's increased intake of high calories and lack of exercise. Children in the last few decades have more access to fast food, especially sugary drinks and high-fat foods. These foods are highly advertised on TV, in magazines, and on billboards. They are easily obtainable. Quick foods and high-caloric snacks are often given to children as rewards for good behavior or as a controlling behavior. Parents' work schedules and after-school activities make fast food a convenient option for meals. Many families do not eat together but are having meals on the run. Social gatherings often have large amounts of food as the focus of the activity. Portion sizes have increased for fast food over the last few decades, resulting in higher caloric intake.

Compounding the rise of convenient, inexpensive, and high-caloric foods is the decrease in activity for most children. Whereas children used to walk to school, now 50 percent of families drive their children, often because of safety, work times, or longer distances. Many schools have cut physical education programs, and private sports teams may be expensive or not in the child's neighborhood. Children may have decreased outside activity based on safety factors or lack of neighborhood parks and play areas. Many children are latchkey kids who are told to stay inside until a parent is home. Gaming, videos, and TV watching have increased and account for a large amount of sedentary time. Many children have inadequate sleep time and are too tired to join an activity.

Social factors play into the above causes of childhood

obesity. Many families lack knowledge of healthy eating and activity lifestyles. The adults in the house are children's role models, and they set the standards for food preferences, amount of intake, willingness to try new foods, and activities that burn calories. Parents may have a lack of knowledge of health risks or be in denial of their own medical issues. I have found that many of these families are simply unaware of healthy behaviors. Several of these factors seems to have contributed to Halley's obesity.

Many families feel that their children will outgrow the "baby fat," or that the weight is genetic or is hormone abnormal-ity–based. However, it is unusual for obese children to have a hormonal etiology for their weight. Rare genetic disorders or thyroid or insulin disease can be eliminated by physical exam and blood tests. The cause of obesity in children involves the individual's metabolism, which is determined by intake, level of exercise, and some genetic predisposition.

Factors such as body types, like stocky or willowy, and muscle versus fat weight must be considered but may be only significant for the slightly overweight child. The BMI may not be helpful for some children because of the changing body shape or for athletic children with large muscle mass. Diagnosis is precise with methods used in research such as bioelectric impedance analysis and underwater weighing to assess fat percentage. These are not practical for a clinic setting. If the BMI seems inaccurate for a child, skinfold thickness and waist circumference are easy to measure.

COMPLICATIONS OF OBESITY

Physicians and other professionals acknowledge the epidemic effects of obesity on social change and the cost to society. Many health risks are attributable to early obesity. Complications from obesity are increasingly documented in children. The following diagnoses are becoming more common.

Hypertension (high blood pressure) is commonly associated with obesity. Hypertension has no symptoms until extremely high. It is diagnosed during routine exams and school or sports physicals. Long-term hypertension creates stress on heart muscles and frays blood vessels. Elevated blood lipids, such as cholesterol, and elevated blood glucose may be associated with high blood pressure.

Diabetes type 2 is a disease that affects the body's processing of glucose sugar. The child's body is resistant to insulin, a hormone that carries glucose into a cell. I have seen this disease increasing in children as the obesity epidemic increases and as children consume more carbohydrates and overload glucose in the bloodstream. The cell rejects carrying of too much glucose into the cell for energy.

Forty percent of children with diabetes type 2 may have no symptoms until the disease has progressed. Then the child may experience increased thirst and urination, tiredness, blurred vision, and slow healing of infections. Darkened skin near the neck, acanthosis nigrans, is noted in association with diabetes 2.

A serious consequence of obesity and overload of calories is *fatty liver* disease, in which fat accumulates in the liver and causes cellular damage with potential to progression to cirrhosis (dying liver cells) and ultimately to the need for a liver transplant.

I have seen that *asthma* is increasing in children with obesity. The cause is unknown but may be from airflow obstruction in heavy children, inflammation of cells that seems to occur more in overweight children, and an unknown decrease in the usefulness of inhaled steroids. Unfortunately, the child who wheezes is less likely to exercise, thus adding to the obesity problem.

I frequently see *sleep apnea*, which is a disease associated with obesity. We see obese children who have nighttime breathing problems with a decrease in oxygen to the body. Sixty percent of obese children will have snoring and lapses of breathing, sleep disruption, daytime tiredness, and learning problems because of daytime sleepiness and irritability. Sleep apnea with obesity is associated with hypertension, decrease in heart function, large tonsils and adenoids, and decreased airway muscle tone.

Orthopedic problems are of concern in the obese child as the extra weight may create strain on the growing bones of the knees and hips. Many older children complain of knee pain, which may indicate knee damage from carrying the weight or referred pain from the hips. A vicious cycle occurs as the heavy child does not feel like the extra work of exercise, and the lack of movement only adds more pounds. Many overweight children tell me they feel shy during gym or team sports and will defer playing whenever possible.

Hormonal diseases associated with obesity are quite rare. They may be suspected if there is a strong family history of thyroid or adrenal problems. Low thyroid levels occur when the thyroid gland is underactive and lowers the basic rate of metabolism in the body. Symptoms in the child may be tiredness, feeling cold, constipation, a hoarse voice, and dry skin. Excess adrenal hormones are extremely rare; symptoms are excess body hair, ease of bruising, and muscle weakness. I suspect these illnesses in an obese child if the heart rate is slow as in a low thyroid or blood pressure is high in a child with high adrenal hormones. Early puberty in obese children has been considered a consequence of obesity. There have not been definitive studies to prove this as the age of puberty has been decreasing prior to the obesity epidemic.

The *psychological impact* of obesity in children ranges from harassment, intimidation, bullying, low self-esteem, exclusion from social groups to unconscious bias or outright discrimination by teachers. These experiences may often be traumatic, not only impacting the child's learning, but also resulting in long-term psychological consequences. Out of frustration and anxiety, the child may further isolate himself or herself and resort to eating more food for comfort. Children may be reticent to participate in class discussions or may be too tired, thus decreasing their learning potentials.

TREATMENT OF OBESITY

I have found that the measurement of height and weight alone on growth curves are helpful to screen for the need to further assess the child. Triceps skinfold tests may be helpful but are difficult to do accurately. The best assessment is the BMI. It is calculated from a formula (weight in kilograms divided by square of the height in meters) but is easily looked up on a smartphone or on the internet. For a child, "overweight" means being over 85 percent, and "obese" means being over 95 percent on the correct chart. For adults, the BMI correlates with the amount of subcutaneous and total body fat, blood pressure measurements, and lipid blood levels. Because children have healthy blood vessels, the correlation is not clear. However, the number can act as a goal to help families.

Diet is culturally and economically based. Today many busy families depend on fast food as a cheap and quick way to obtain meals. Media promotes special deals on pizzas and fried fast food that are usually high in carbohydrates and saturated oils. Many poor neighborhoods with limited public transportation have minimal access to stores with fresh fruits and vegetables. School lunches are notorious for being high in carbohydrates and fat! Some schools across the United States are now planning gardens and advocating for changes in the lunches, thanks in part to Michele Obama's influence. Recently there has been more research on dietary changes for heart protection.

These findings can be translated into help with food intake for the obese child and her or his family.

The ideal Mediterranean diet of fish, fruits, vegetables, and whole-grain bread requires careful planning, shopping, and preparing. In addition, food products have changed significantly in the last few decades. Portion sizes in restaurants have increased. Many packaged foods have a considerable amount of high-fructose corn syrup in the product, adding calories and affecting insulin function. Many beverages have added sugar. These sugar-laden drinks are part of some of the fast-food specials that flood the advertising media.

Media reports have recently advised a ketogenic or keto diet for weight loss. This diet requires eliminating carbohydrates (foods that contain any grains or sugars, such as bread, pasta, rice, and desserts). Instead of using glucose as a source of energy in the brain, the cells use ketones, which are found in fats. Fat in the body is converted to ketones for use in the brain, and body weight is decreased. Adults on this diet describe a feeling of change in their thinking. Some children with seizures are successfully treated with the ketogenic diet. However, this diet is currently not advised for treatment of childhood obesity.

We know that socioeconomic factors may also hamper a recommended exercise program. Many inner-city neighborhoods without yards are not safe for playing, and areas for sports may be lacking. Parks may not be easily accessible. Equipment for play may be lacking for some schools. Most after-school sports activities require a fee and a uniform, and thus many families are unable to participate. Suburban life affects exercise as the culture is automobile based. Children are often driven to school and to planned activities. Fear is prevalent if a child runs or bicycles without adult supervision.

The culture of staying indoors with television, gaming, and other electronics adds to the pattern of inactivity. Even at restaurants children are often seen focusing on their cell phone apps rather than conversing with others. Many children in the grade-school-age range spend more hours gaming than doing homework or interacting with their families. These activities may affect psychosocial development and contribute to an increase in eating snack food and decreasing of any physical movement activity.

Families often hope there will be a quick way for the child to lose the pounds. Unfortunately, there are no magic medications to melt away the pounds. Surgical procedures are not approved for children due to lack of research and ethical issues as these procedures can rarely be reversed. Successful programs to help obese children lose and keep off weight always have four components. These are modification of diet with restriction of calories, an exercise program that is realistic for the child and family, behavior modification education about food choices, and portion control. Of course family members must be willing to modify long-standing habits.

Pharmacological research in drugs for weight loss shows limited success. There are two newly FDA-approved drugs for appetite suppression, Lorcaserin and phentermine/topiramate. As drug research is rare in children, these may not be available for some years for the pediatric population. There is one drug that has been minimally studied, Orlistat, which works by decreasing fat absorption. However, the drug has potential side effects, such as urgent, frequent, and loose bowel movements, and it is not advised for children.

The drug metformin has been used to improve insulin sensitivity so that insulin can carry the needed glucose into the cell if diabetes type 2 cannot be controlled. If lipid blood levels are very high, the drug clofibrate has been used.

Antioxidants have been ineffective in weight loss. If liver enzymes are seriously elevated, as in fatty liver, a hepato-protective (liver protective) drug, such as ursodeoxychotic acid, has been prescribed by liver specialists.

Success may be achieved for obese children if there is a multidisciplinary group approach including providers with interests in obesity issues, health educators, dietitians, physical fitness specialists, and therapists. Unfortunately, insurance companies usually do not cover health education visits. Because the issue of obesity in children is becoming epidemic, it may be possible to obtain grant money for a clinical trial. Ideally, there would be weekly visits with the above specialists, group visits with other families, weight checks, grocery store buying classes, and outreach for entire families to become involved.

FOLLOW-UP FOR HALLEY, THREE MONTHS LATER

Initially Halley's mother is reticent to show concern regarding her daughter's weight. However, Halley's aunt has recently been diagnosed with diabetes type 2 and requires insulin shots. Halley's aunt's liver enzymes had been elevated but have dropped to normal with only a 5 percent weight loss. After talking with the aunt and several other friends, the mother agreed to have Halley, her brother, her father, and herself attend some classes regarding the complications of obesity and prevention measures. They soon realize this is a family issue as each person has some form of fast food daily and an inactive lifestyle. The family is surprised to see their values on a BMI chart, which show them to be in a dangerously obese range. Halley is excited to be planning some fun outings. And after some playful teasing, she decided she would try a vegetable a day! They have weigh-in visits weekly. At the three-month period, they have all lost significant weight and report that they feel more invigorated and active.

Lifestyle changes rock!

RESOURCES FOR FAMILIES

- Https://www.healthiergeneration.org provides guidance regarding talking to children about food changes.
- Https://www.obesitymedicine.org lists many resources for families with obese children.
- Https://ihcw.aap.org/, the Institute for Healthy Childhood Weight, is established for pediatric obesity prevention, assessment, and treatment.
- Https://healthykidshealthyfuture.org provides help regarding eating better, getting kids moving, and limiting screen time.

CHAPTER 7

Tomas: An Eight-Year-Old with
Learning Differences

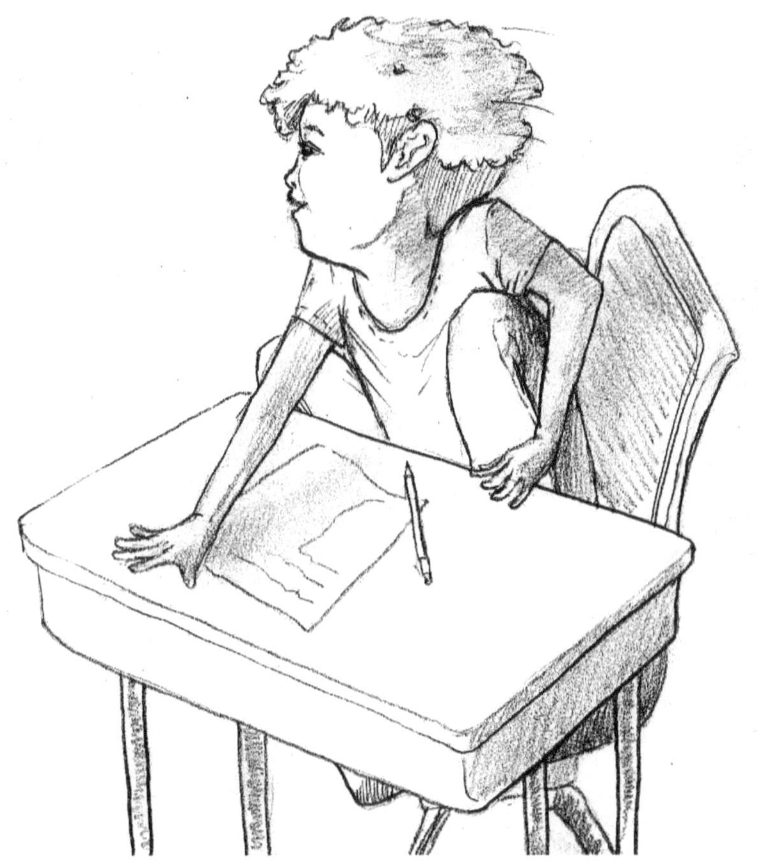

Tomas

TOMAS'S father recently called me to discuss a school conference with Tomas's teacher. He tells me that his teacher is very concerned that Tom may have a learning disability. I will use the term "learning differences" instead of "learning disabilities" as I believe all students are unique, and some learn at different rates and styles from their peers.

Tomas's father says that he can hardly read his son's handwriting and that Tomas cannot keep his numbers in a straight line on the page. He is disorganized with his homework and often loses it or forgets to hand it in. He seems different from his siblings and friends his age. Tomas is able to beat them with complex video games, but he has never matched them in schoolwork. He is clumsy in group sports and prefers solo sports, like riding his bike or swimming. "We feel Tomas is a great kid, but he is falling behind."

Recently Tomas has become frustrated and breaks his pencils and wads up his papers. He does not want to hang out with his friends. He has recent nightmares and has decreased appetite. His teacher is concerned that Tomas is being teased by other students about his schoolwork. His father is worried that Tomas's self-esteem is becoming diminished. Tomas recently said, "I want to disappear. I can't do anything right." Dad says the school wants to give Tomas an IEP, but he is worried that this will label him and follow him forever. He is also concerned that he might be teased or bullied.

Tomas's other father is also concerned, but he thinks Tomas will grow out of the school difficulties. They have been reading about suicide in young children and would like him to see a therapist about his self-esteem. I advise Tomas's fathers to bring him into clinic. I explain I am concerned about a possible learning difference and low self-image.

I tell them that the physical exam may give me a clue to his problems. Different learning styles are by far the most common culprits. However, any child with learning differences should be evaluated for any medical causes, especially hearing or vision problems. A child who does not hear or see well may try to get clues about schoolwork from copying from other children. The child may not be aware that his or her hearing or vision is different from others. All children want to fit in, and they will try to compensate in some way for the deficit. Children with dyslexia and other reading problems will try to figure out the stories by listening to other children and studying the illustrations. Tomas's father says his reading level is average and that his handwriting and his math columns are the main issues. Both his fathers suspect that he is much smarter than his work shows.

Genetics play a major role regarding learning differences. As Tomas is an adopted child, comparison with blood relatives is not possible. They do not have information about the pregnancy with regards to drugs or illness. They do know that Tomas had a normal birth history and has had no major illnesses, injuries, or medications.

THE CLINIC VISIT

Tomas appears to be a healthy and robust child who responds well to questions and the exam. Fortunately, his vision and hearing screens are normal. He has no abnormal facial or body characteristics that might indicate a medical syndrome. His physical exam is normal, including a careful neurological exam for muscle coordination and reflexes.

I ask Tomas about his friends and how he likes school. He says he is being teased a lot by his classmates. He mumbles that "I don't want to be around anymore." I explain to him about the differences everyone has in learning some things. Some of his classmates are great at drawing, some play the piano, some run really fast, some read older-age books, but all of them are less skilled in other ways. For example, the piano player has problems with subtraction, and the artist has problems with spelling.

I ask Tomas to play a few games with pencil and paper, such as printing his name, copying a trapezoid, copying a line with an end pointing out like an arrow, and a stick figure of a person. Tomas hesitates and says, "I can't copy corners, but I will try." Next I ask him to to draw a circle, write his name inside the circle, and then cut out the circle. He willingly tries with each task but is unable to copy the work or cut the circle. Of interest, he is able to describe the shapes: "That's a two-headed arrow. That's a lopsided rectangle." He is able to read a sentence in an age-appropriate book without problems. During these games he remains on focus without any extraneous movements.

I discuss the potential of Tomas having a learning difference. He has issues with fine motor coordination and visual motor perception. He has problems in transferring what he sees into signals for his fingers to execute the shapes. He has an excellent vocabulary and reading ability. Fortunately, Tomas has excellent focus and the willingness to try hard at the testing games.

LEARNING DIFFERENCES

Learning differences are neurologically based processing problems that can affect different tracts in the brain. There are several common learning differences.

Visual Perceptional or Motor or Visual-Motor Problems

This is a disorder of misunderstanding information about what they see and their abilities to copy or draw. As with Tomas, these children have a hard time copying shapes or words, holding a pencil, or using scissors. Children who cannot copy directions from the board with a pencil may be able to use a keyboard, which involves a different nerve tract. Time, maturity, and special tutoring are very helpful for these children. Tomas fits into this category.

AUDITORY PROCESSING DISORDER

This disorder includes problems with differences in the sound of words, the order of words, the interpretation of these sounds. It is compounded by background noises. The children have problems following directions and remembering what they learned.

CLASSIC DYSLEXIA

This defines the child with word or letter reversals. It is a visual-processing disorder. There are many tutoring styles that include using a finger to write in the air, sounding out the vowels, or printing in the sand or salt to get the pattern of letter sequence. Using a window cut in blank paper to isolate the word may help.

ATTENTION ISSUES

A child with learning differences may also have an attention disorder with or without hyperactivity. If the learning differences are addressed and tutoring is helpful to give the child some strategies to compensate for his or her problem, the child becomes more focused in the classroom. Natural maturity may come around age nine or ten years, and the children will usually improve their focus and increase their calmness.

THE ISSUE OF GAMING

Tomas's fathers are worried that he spends too much time playing video games. This is an area of success for Tomas. They are torn in their decisions regarding the amount of time he plays. Our children have grown up in a rapidly evolving electronic age. Keyboarding, oral directions to AI (artificial intelligence), CDs, DVDs, and gaming will be a significant part of their lives for academics, careers, avocations, and leisure activities. As happens with all social changes, it can be difficult to maintain a balance for physical and mental health.

Of course limits are reasonable. However, there are some pluses to gaming. For a child with visual motor dysfunction, the neurological stimulus may help the child to coordinate brain signals with fine-motor muscles. Because Tomas must respond to a visual signal with fine-motor hand movement, this neurological pathway is reenforced. Some children who are electronic gamers have improved their copying, writing, and drawing.

We are all aware of the violence depicted in many games. However, there are many strategy games that may be played with other children that involve intellectual planning, calculations, memory, and cooperation, especially games which have the child create cities and cultures.

THE ISSUE OF SCHOOL REGULATIONS AND SCHOOL HELP FOR THE CHILD WITH LD

I discuss with Tomas's fathers the frustration they may experience with the school system. Cities, counties, and states vary widely regarding timing and availability of testing, regulations for program eligibility, availability of expert tutors, changes in the classroom environment and in teaching style so that each child understands directions, and expectations for her or his schoolwork. I explain that some families find a local support group that can guide them on the legal rights of a child with an LD.

PSYCHOLOGICAL ISSUES FOR CHILDREN WITH LDS

Suicide is a serious concern for young children who have risk factors, some of which are schoolwork problems or learning differences. Suicide is the third leading cause of death in twelve-year-old children. One in eight children between ages six and twelve have had suicidal thoughts. Males complete suicide four times more than females, but females attempt the act three times more than males.

Risk factors for suicide in young children are recent loss of family or home, underlying mental illness, lack of social support, disruption in the family, a traumatic event, and school issues. LDs and ADD/ADHD are significant risk factors. Decease in school performance is common.

Warning signs may be very subtle in the young child. Decrease in appetite and sleeping problems may be mild. Withdrawal from friends and family is common. Feelings of sadness and hopelessness are often difficult to ascertain. Some children have a preoccupation with death and will write and draw scenes about suicide. It is crucial that a therapist or family member talk directly to the child and ask about feelings of self-harm. If the child with LD or attention issues receives therapy and tutoring, feelings of low self-worth will decrease.

FOLLOW-UP FOR TOMAS

An IEP helps Tomas's family and teacher understand that he is a very intelligent boy with excellent understanding of verbal directions, reading, comprehension, and math. His problem is defined by visual-motor disability. His learning issue is improved with tutoring and learning hints such as using graph paper for lining up numbers and always using lined paper. He practices making letters in the air with his index finger, starting with large movements and then narrowing the movements to train the muscles to remember the movements involved in making the letters. Fortunately his school and his teacher take his testing result of LD very seriously and attempt to use the suggestions from his tutor.

I tell Tomas that fortunately we live in an era of electronic communication so that in time he can learn to use a keyboard and printer as he advances through the grades. I also tell him and his family that I expect he will succeed in school. After several tutoring and therapy sessions, his mood improves, and he feels more in control of his schoolwork

Many adults have found that they can be successful without legible handwriting.

Like doctors!

RESOURCES FOR PARENTS

- Https://ldaamerica.org/parents/—Learning Disabilities Association of America—provides information with articles and booklets for each type of LD.
- Https://www.parentcenterhub.org/parentgroups/ is a center that gives parents information and resources.
- Https://www.helpguide.org/articles/autism-learning-disabilities/helping-children-with-learning-disabilities.htm provides education and suggestions with emphasis on advocating at the school as legal issues, complex regulations, and lack of resources evolve.

CHAPTER 8

Marcus: A Six-Year-Old with Recurrent Abdominal Pain and Social Isolation

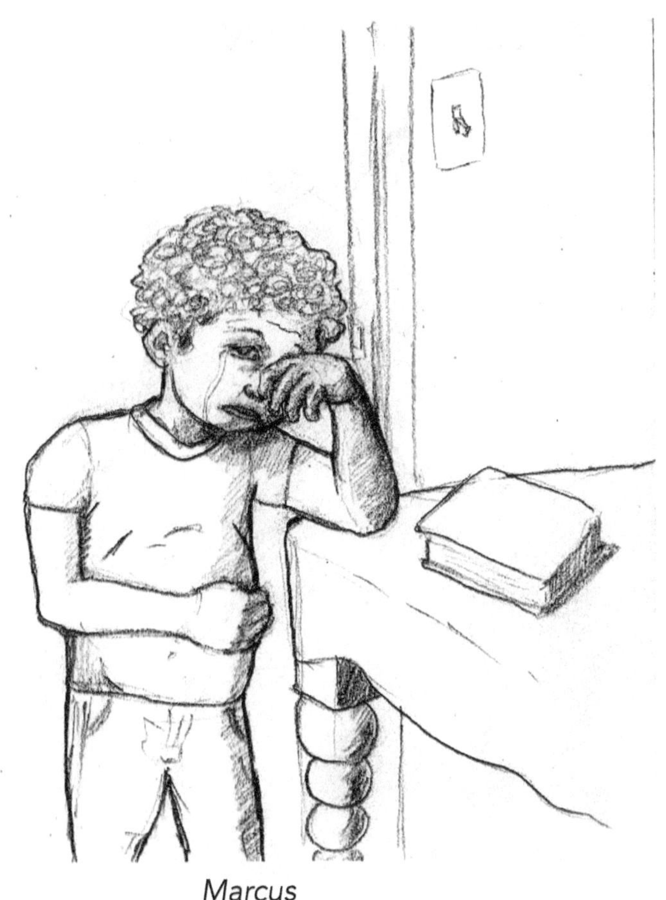

Marcus

MARCUS'S mother contacts me regarding his recurrent episodes of abdominal pain. These pains occur for a few days every month over the last two years. She is now concerned as he is missing school and becoming irritable. Prior to these episodes, he was an active healthy boy. At first she thought he was just acting out and exaggerating, but now he seems more upset. She contacts me, and I advise that they come into clinic.

During our clinic visit, Marcus describes his pain as, "around my belly button," and, "all the time." His mother says he does not have fever, weight loss, pain waking him at night, vomiting, or any problem with diarrhea. Marcus says he can "pee" and "poo" okay. His mother says that he rarely goes, "number 2," and sometimes he has stool or smearing on his underwear. His classmates tease him when they smell his accidents. He does not seem to be aware of his bowel leakage. Marcus's teacher is suggesting to the mother than he may have a serious psychological problem. His mother disagrees and states there are no problems other than the pain. Marcus agrees that his only "tummy" symptom is pain.

His mother is worried because his aunt has regional enteritis (Crohn's disease), a serious autoimmune disease with intestinal symptoms. She is worried he may have inherited this from his aunt.

Marcus's physical exam reveals to me a healthy-appearing boy whose height and weight are in the normal range. He does not appear stressed, pale, or ill in any way. But his abdomen seems somewhat distended. When I pressed on his abdomen, there was no discomfort. He says okay to a rectal exam, which reveals a large amount of stool. Marcus's mother agrees to an X-ray, which shows copious stool throughout the intestines.

Marcus's mother is surprised by the obvious diagnosis of constipation. Listening to the discussion, Marcus interrupts, saying, "But I don't have to go."

CONSTIPATION IN CHILDREN

Over my years as a pediatrician, I have noted that constipation is the most common cause of recurrent abdominal pain presenting in a pediatric office. Children often do not respond to the body's signals that it is time "to go." A trip to the bathroom may interrupt their current activities or embarrass them in front of their peers. The sensations then pass. The child forgets to make a bowel movement on his or her returning home. Stool builds up and stretches the intestinal walls, causing a malfunction of the nerve signals that signal the presence of stool. These children actually do not feel the sensation that they need to move their bowels. The family may not suspect constipation as there may be overflow stool coming out.

The sensation may occasionally cease completely and cause the inability for the child to move stool voluntarily. The intestinal nerves that signal that stool is present are damaged by the stretching of the intestinal walls. As this occurs, there may be an uncontrollable overflow of liquid stool on the underwear. This problem of severe retention and resultant overflow is called encopresis, a condition that causes significant psychosocial problems at home and school.

Parents often feel there must be more medical problems than encopresis. They often request that I order more testing. Marcus's mother is especially concerned about the family history of regional enteritis, Crohn's disease. These concerns will usually resolve when the pain and soiling resolve.

CONSTIPATION TREATMENT

My goal of treatment for severe constipation is to achieve a return of muscle tone. It is necessary to clean out the intestinal passageway so the pressure on the muscles is decreased. One effective treatment is the use of oral polyethylene glycol at a maximum dose for a few days. Some children are comfortable using a few days of enemas to provide rapid relief of pain. Daily oral use of the polyethylene glycol or a form of the mineral magnesium is usually advised. These are found in any drugstore or health store. These are usually taken for several months to allow the muscle tone and the nerve signals to recover. Marcus and his family can determine what dose of medication results in normal stool passage and does not cause diarrhea.

Dietary changes—including more foods with fiber, more water intake—and a schedule for daily bowel movement will maintain intestinal muscle tone. Scheduling a time for a bowel movement in the morning before school will ensure he or she will not have the need to suppress the signal of stool and not have accidents. The family needs to be on guard to make sure the pattern of withholding stool does not recur.

Most families have found that family therapy may help with the child's sense of shame, self-esteem, and worries about being taunted at school. Ideally the child's local clinic or hospital may have some children's groups where they can share their experiences and not feel so isolated.

DISEASES CAUSING ABDOMINAL PAIN OTHER THAN CONSTIPATION

Diagnosing recurrent abdominal pain is often not as straightforward as with Marcus and his period of constipation and encopresis. Frequent complaints of abdominal pain create a difficult issue for the pediatric provider and the family. Some studies show that 10 percent of school-age children may complain frequently of stomachaches. Many visits to the clinic result in loss of school attendance and parental employment.

These challenges are formidable for all parties. Testing for a serious condition is time-consuming and expensive. Treatment options for the management of the common causes are often difficult to follow. The psychosocial component for the families may be complex.

Serious diagnoses are rare. When the symptoms or findings on physical exam are suspected, a diagnosis such as a tumor, an anatomic problem of malformed intestines, a chronic infection, an inflammatory disease such as colitis, esophageal reflux, or in females, ovarian or uterine problems may be suspected.

These symptoms do not normally occur with constipation:

- Weight loss without decreased food intake
- Increase in height less than peers' growth
- Frequent vomiting
- Chronic diarrhea
- Blood in vomit or stool
- Persistent pain in one area
- Fevers without obvious cause
- Abdominal lump
- Family history of bowel disease, like ulcerative colitis or regional enteritis
- Heartburn (reflux) with or without pain
- Urinary problems such as pain or bleeding with urination
- Associated skin or joint problems that flare when the abdominal pain recurs

CAUSES OF THE SERIOUS DISEASES

Infections may cause abdominal pain in children. Usually there is diarrhea with blood and mucous, but occasionally there may only be pain. Bacteria such as campylobacter, salmonella, shigella. and some E. coli types may cause irritation and diarrhea. Infection may also be caused by helicobacter pylori, an intestinal bacteria that causes irritation of the stomach lining and ulcers. Parasitic infections also cause irritation and diarrhea. Usually there is a family history of travel, a relative or friend who travels, or a known outbreak in a community. An exception would be the parasite giardia, which is found in the streams of the Sierra Mountains in California. These infections are transmitted by infected food, inadequate hygiene, unsafe drinking water, and poor handwashing.

Issues about *gluten* intake and sensitivity are common, especially in the current media. Gluten is composed of proteins found in wheat flour. The autoimmune disease known as celiac sprue is caused by the body's immune system. In the presence of gluten, the immune cells start attacking and damaging the villi of the small intestine. These intestinal villi become flattened and are unable to absorb nutrients, causing poor digestion and in severe cases, malnutrition. Less common than celiac sprue is an allergic reaction to gluten with hives and a feeling of constriction in the throat. Sensitivity to gluten is suspected when the family has a vague feeling that "The child does better off wheat products." Unfortunately, many families wrongly think their children have celiac and keep them off foods containing wheat flour. The child is not allowed to eat many popular foods—like bread, pasta, pizza, cookies, and cake—or any food with possible gluten. Most providers will suggest that formal testing by blood and endoscopy be performed to establish the disease.

Liver disease causing abdominal pain is suspected when the liver is enlarged or the child is jaundiced (yellowing of the skin and eyes). The child may have an inherited liver disease, been exposed to a hepatitis virus, or has a reaction to certain over-the-counter or prescription medications. The discomfort of liver disease usually is constant and progressively increases.

Kidney disease may cause abdominal or back pain. There may be blood and/or protein in the urine. Families may have concern about an inherited kidney disease. The causes of these diseases are rare and complex. Usually a child with abdominal pain is screened with a urine test, which will indicate if further testing is needed.

Families may fear *cancer* when their child has abdominal discomfort. Fortunately, intestinal tumors are rare in children. A tumor may be suspected by the provider or a family member feeling a lump, noticing weight loss in the child, or increasing localized pain.

Ulcerative colitis, celiac sprue (as discussed previously), and regional enteritis are *inflammatory autoimmune diseases*. Symptoms of these diseases are caused by the child's own white blood cells (lymphocytes) in the immune system attack the child's intestinal cells, causing pain, diarrhea, and blood in the stools. The intestinal cells are made up of villi, which become flattened when attacked by the lymphocytes and cannot absorb nutrients. Children with an autoimmune disease may have fevers, weight loss, and below average height compared to growth charts and/or skin or joint manifestations.

TESTING FOR THESE DISEASES

Laboratory blood tests are often ordered by a pediatric provider to check for infection or anemia from blood loss, and to screen for bacterial antibodies, gluten sensitivity, liver disease, kidney function, and inflammation. Urine may be tested for infection or decreased function of the kidneys. Stool may be tested for blood, infection by bacteria or parasites, or fat that is not being absorbed.

Tumors or cysts may be felt in the abdomen by the pediatric provider. An ultrasound or a CT scan will determine the next steps. Decision of which imaging test is based on size and location and other findings found on the physical examination.

A child may need an endoscopy, sigmoidoscopy, or colonoscopy procedure to diagnose an intestinal disease. Proof of celiac involves a biopsy of the small intestine. An anesthesiologist sedates the child, and a gastroenterologist, a physician specializing in intestines and other abdominal organs, inserts a small tube with a light, camera, and tiny clippers into the esophagus, then the stomach, and then into the small intestine, where a biopsy is performed. Proof of ulcerative colitis or regional enteritis is done with a sigmoidoscopy or colonoscopy done as above but into the lower intestines via the rectum.

These screening tests help the provider know what further evaluation is needed. Treatment is different for each diagnosis. The huge number of abdominal diagnoses are beyond the scope of this book.

NEW RESEARCH

Research has recently focused on the complex interaction between the intestinal nerves and the brain's central nervous system. For decades, recurrent abdominal pain in children had been thought to be caused by motility (movement of the intestinal muscles) problems, leading to constipation and psychosocial problems, as in Marcus's case. Today it is thought that some children have an exaggerated pain response to abdominal pressure. Neurohormones such as serotonin and dopamine are known to reside in the intestine and are thought to affect digestion and motility. An imbalance of neurohormones may cause intestinal inflammation.

Recently there is an increased interest in the intestinal biome. This microbiome is an intestinal bacterial and fungal community harboring both healthy and unhealthy organisms. Tens of trillions of organisms of one thousand species account for ten times more than cells found in the total human body. Current genetic testing and identification of organisms and their correlation with intestinal symptoms is now under research.

The intestines of those children with inflammatory bowel diseases such as ulcerative colitis and regional enteritis have been found to sometimes have differing organisms from those without disease. The evaluation of the microbiome is currently only done by researchers and not in clinics. Current thinking is that there may be a correlation with the intestinal neurohormones and the intestine microbiome comprised of organisms.

Regarding treatment options, biofeedback has been used in some gastroenterology clinics to help the child learn to use their sphincters (the strip of muscle that holds or releases the stool in the lower colon) correctly. The child has a tiny pressure sensor in the lower intestine that shows a visual reward on the screen when he or she learns to tighten or relax the internal sphincters to allow stool to move along and coordinate with the external sphincter. The children love this video game style set up.

Some families have been treating the intestinal biome by giving probiotics, which are "good" organisms, especially when the child has been given antibiotics that decrease the normal intestinal flora. Healthy organisms are found in kefir and yogurt, kimchi, sauerkraut, kombucha, miso, sourdough. Probiotics are also available in drugstores and health food stores.

REVISIT WITH MARCUS

Marcus's family agrees with the diagnosis of constipation and encopresis and wish to forgo any further testing unless the pain persists or new symptoms occur. Marcus returns to our clinic and says he is willing to keep drinking the polyethylene glycol every evening. Initially he resisted getting up early and trying to have a bowel movement before school. But as he begins to have "clean" days at school and to have increased sensation in his rectum that stool is present, he agrees to keep trying. Unfortunately, his family was not successful in encouraging him to eat more vegetables with fiber. After a month, they stop the medicine, and some signs of constipation recur. After some experimentation, Marcus and his family find an amount of the polyethylene glycol that results in easily passing stool without dry, hard stools or diarrhea. This family feels they are on the right track for understanding the complexity of a child's growth and development, and that Marcus has learned a lot. He is now accepted among his peers at school, and his teacher and parents are pleased!

Success!

RESOURCES FOR FAMILIES

- Https://childmind.org/search/?fwp_term=encopresis is a site with clear discussions of encopresis for families.
- Https://www.aafp.org/afp/2018/0615/p785.html is a site with good discussion of abdominal pain in children.
- Https://pedsinreview.aappublications.org/content/36/9/392 is a scholarly article on abdominal pain in children.

CHAPTER 9

Chloe: A Five-Year-Old Girl with Sexualized Behaviors

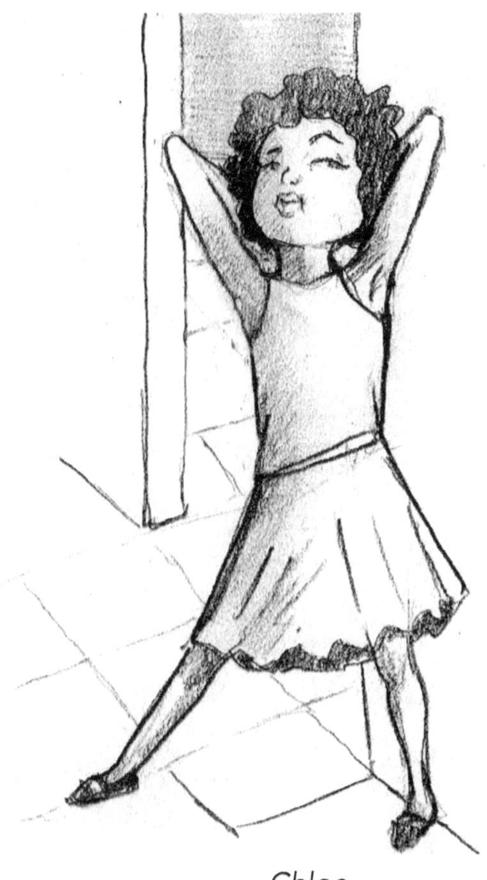

Chloe

CHLOE'S mother calls me about her concern that Chloe has been acting in a sexual manner in her classroom. Chloe had been a quiet, curious, gentle child until a few weeks ago, when her teacher sensed a change in her. Recently, Chloe seems more easily upset and cries frequently. She starts conflicts with her friends and often swears at them. During recess she pulls down her pants and underwear and wiggles her whole body in a suggestive manner. Chloe has not participated recently in class or finished her homework. When questioned about her behaviors, she responds that she doesn't understand.

The mother tells me the teacher recently asked the parents and a therapist to attend a meeting to discuss Chloe's behaviors and changes. In the meeting, the teacher describes how Chloe has been acting. She suggests that Chloe should have some visits with the therapist. The mother concurs, saying she is concerned about the change in her daughter. Chloe's father says, "I'm shocked. My daughter would not do that. I don't want a record made of this."

The therapist asks the family if there have been any changes in the home, like new persons, moves, employment changes, illness or any issues in family, babysitters, neighborhood, or friends who have contact with Chloe. She asks about who is living in the home and if anyone has an addiction or mental illness problem. Chloe's father becomes upset and says he feels he is being accused and walks out of the meeting. His wife remains silent but follows him a few paces behind.

The schoolteachers and the therapist agree that Chloe's behavior is not age appropriate. By the age of five most boys and girls are aware of the social norms regarding their bodies and behaviors in a school or other social environment. These professionals are very concerned for Chloe as the behaviors are inappropriate for her age and that her schoolwork and her peer interactions are being affected. The school professionals decide they will write a letter requesting a return meeting to discuss Chloe's behavior.

Meanwhile her parents are able to concur that their daughter needs some help. They agree that Chloe might benefit from seeing a therapist. I see Chloe in our clinic after her meetings with the therapist. I explain that I am worried that someone might have touched her "privates". We draw some pictures with crayons about what she tells the therapist. She agrees to let me look at her "privates". She appears to have no damage to her genitals.

After several weeks of therapy, Chloe begins to trust the professional therapist, and she talks about her babysitter's thirteen-year-old friend, Nicholas. He has offered to teach Chloe video games while the babysitter studies. After a few fun games, he starts showing her pornographic films. She does not wish to watch, but he tells her little girls like it and that they will feel "funny". When she says she wants to ask her mom, he says he will hurt her mom if Chloe talks. Over the next few visits, he does play some video games with her as a cover, but also starts to touch her genitals. Nicholas tells her this is all part of their special "secret".

Though she tells her therapist, Chloe is still frightened that her mother will be hurt. She seems confused and angry. The therapist reassures her that Nicholas will never come over again or harm her or her mother. The family, the boy's parents, and child protective services are contacted. He and his family will be evaluated and treated to find the root of his mental issues.

NORMAL CHILDHOOD DEVELOPMENT

Development is quite variable regarding sexual development and interest in the other gender. The following list of age-appropriate behaviors may be off by years in some children. A child may show sexualized behaviors due to mental illness or hormonal imbalance. Teachers are trained to note the change in sexualized behaviors in a previously well-balanced child. If the behaviors are pathological, they will persist and escalate. There will be other nonsexual clues to a real problem, such as a new emotional imbalance, concern by adults about the actions, possible parental denial, and poor academic school performance. The child may show new behaviors of hyperactivity or of withdrawal and shyness.

Children are naturally curious, especially about their bodies or behaviors they may have seen or experienced. If serious, the developmental stages outlined below may be shifted. Chloe is showing that her development and sexual awareness have been altered.

Note that some children may vary in their staging. A trained therapist will be able to identify if an outlying phase of development for a child is not serious. Some children are unusual in temperament or personality. The child's behavior may be innocent. As long as the behaviors do not include violence, negative sexual words, harm, or control, they may not indicate immediate cause for concern.

AGE-APPROPRIATE BEHAVIORS

Years of age and awareness:

- 2–2.5: Awareness of their own and others' genitalia
- 3–4: Showing, looking, and touching their own and others' bodies

- 5: Becoming more modest and asking for privacy with dressing, bathing, and toileting
- 6: Beginning to ask about how babies are made
- 7: Showing less interest in bodies
- 8: Starting to have some hidden experimentation
- 9: Exchanging information and wishing to read books about development
- 10: Beginning to have interest in the opposite sex

Behaviors at any age that are signs of a problem:

- Behaviors out of the ordinary for the developmental stage
- Frequent and persistent use of sexual language
- Exhibition of genitalia
- Inappropriate physical boundaries
- Preoccupation with sexual actions
- Sexual aggression to other children, adults, or animals, especially if done with control
- Changes in style choices and dress
- Nightmares and new fears
- Fear of places that had been comfortable before
- Fear of certain older children or adults
- Unusual behaviors, even if positive, around some persons
- Paradoxical behavior of overaffectionate behavior focused on the abuser. An abused child may try to please the abuser or to draw attention away from him or her as the bad guy.

If these behaviors are frequent, sexual abuse must be considered. All children will occasionally exhibit behaviors that are odd, but unless there is persistence or escalation, there may be no pathology. Often families or teachers will overreact, which is confusing to the child. Openness and factual age-appropriate discussion will usually result in the truth. Remember that children often do odd behaviors for attention and that children are naturally curious.

My experience is that parents often deny that their child is inappropriate, especially if they are aware of issues at home. They often say, "My child would not do that." "Oh, I am so embarrassed." "People are overreacting." "I don't want the police involved." "So you are calling my child a molester?" "We handle our own problems." Families are usually very ashamed and feel helpless or unsure what will happen. There is media coverage about child molestation and that misbehavior or involvement of a child is a reflection on the family.

CAUSATIONS FOR A CHILD TO ACT OUT SEXUALLY

If a child has been exposed to pornography at an inappropriate age, she or he may have sexual feelings. Pornographic videos and magazines are present in many homes and may not be secured. Children are curious and will try to find hidden items. Children at preschool- and early-grade-school age are at a cuddly stage and welcome benign touches and hugging. If their genitals have been stimulated by action or by images, they may confuse the cuddling and hugging with sexual contact.

Most children have access to electronic media and are curious about portrayals involving sexual language and play. They may ask what words in a current song mean, what a magazine cover means, or why they cannot go to certain movies. Even with family oversight and electronic blocking, children will find a way. Children are curious!

A child may walk in on adults who are having sexual activity/intercourse and ask curious questions. If answered in an age-appropriate way, such as, "We were tickling each other and being silly in a private way," the child should not be affected. If the adults freak out, the child may be frightened or confused by what they saw. Children need to know which behaviors, like toileting or bathing, are private. If children are forced to watch sexual actions, they will be confused about behaviors and their reactions to the sights.

Disrespectful and sexual attitudes are also confusing to a young child. They may not have had their questions answered in a calm factual way, or they hear talk that is laced with emotional outbursts that allude to sex. Confusion about swear words that allude to sex are common. Often the family member is not aware the child does not know the meaning of many swear words, and the adult becomes upset when the child later uses a sexual word.

Some children become overly sexualized when there is no privacy or body boundaries. Some families are comfortable with nudity and are able to teach their children what is appropriate outside the home. Most grade-school-age children are instinctively private about their bodies. Each child is unique in comprehension, so families must be careful in understanding their children's comfort level.

Sexual abuse at any age results in psychological damage that may be manifested by withdrawal and silence or by physical actions inappropriate for the age. Younger children are affected by acting out sexual behaviors with their peers, whereas older children often become very withdrawn and reticent to communicate. The abusing older child or adult may frighten the child with verbal threats that the family will be hurt if the child tells anyone. Thus the abuse becomes the "dirty little secret" that the child buries in her or his psyche.

TREATMENT FOR THE SEXUALLY ACTING-OUT CHILD

Therapy for the child must be individualized by a therapist with experience in these cases. Every situation and family are unique. The goal of therapy is to identify the source of the acting out, possibly change the living situation, and help the child to understand that he or she is innocent and that the adult is the "bad one." The child may wish to transfer to a different school as he or she may be fearful that "Everyone will know." Children have often been threatened that if they talk, their families will be hurt. It may take many sessions for the children to understand that they and their families will be safe, that they were not at fault, and that they are loved by their families.

FOLLOW-UP FOR CHLOE

Once Chloe has revealed her "secret" to her mother, her behavior improves. She still cries and has some sleep disturbance but is much improved. She is much calmer in school. The other children begin to play with her without referring to her prior behaviors. She gradually resumes her cheerful demeanor. Her family is relieved and happy that they have Chloe back. However, she may have some issues during adolescence.

Children are resilient!

RESOURCES FOR FAMILIES

- The National Child Traumatic Stress organization (https://www.nctsn.org/what-is-child-trauma/trauma-types/sexual-abuse) lists statistics and signs of child sexual abuse and ways of reporting.

- Darkness to Light (https://www.d2l.org/) gives factual information and steps to protect children.
- Https://www.rainn.org/articles/child-sexual-abuse has an excellent summary of child sexual abuse, symptoms and warning signs, and resources for help.

CHAPTER 10

Dione: A Seven-Year-Old with Short Stature

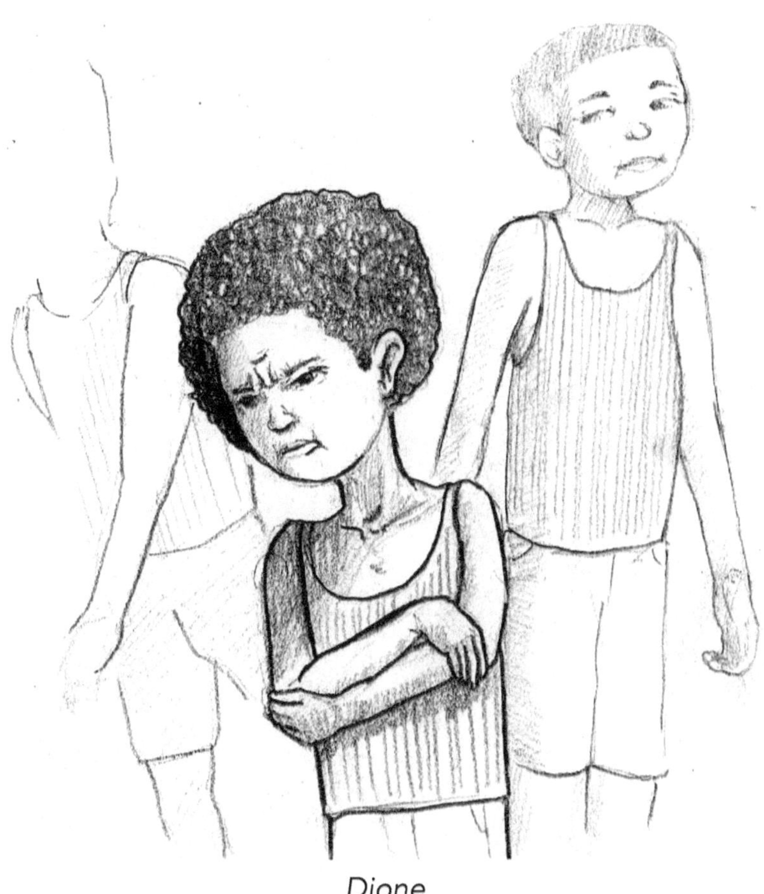

Dione

DIONE is a seven-year-old who comes to our pediatric clinic for the purpose of signing the sports form for his soccer team. His parents feel he is in excellent health and that he is an excellent student. He is interested in and excels in playing all sports. Several of his cousins play basketball at the university level. Dione says that he will be a basketball star when he grows up, and then a team doctor when he gets old!

Dione's parents are concerned that he is the shortest boy in his class. He was a normal-sized infant with no medical problems. He has never had a serious illness other than occasional asthma. He takes his inhaler medications once in a while. When he started preschool, his parents noticed that he was always the shortest boy in his group. The parents appear to be in the middle range for height.

Dione's physical is completely normal except that for the last few years, numbers on his growth chart show that he is shorter than the majority of children his age, and he is shorter than expected considering his parents' heights. Dione's weight is proportional to his height. His growth line is parallel to the average lines, which shows that there was no sudden drop as might happen with an intercurrent illness.

I suggest that Dione's family call me with the names of his asthma medications. I also suggest that they talk to his tall cousins to find out their height history during childhood and at what age they had their growth spurts. A few days later, Dione's parents respond that one of the asthma inhalers is beclomethasone. They were unsure of the frequency of use as he carries it in his backpack. They have texted the cousins and learn that three of the four were the shortest in their classes until a spurt of height in their senior year of high school, and height growth continued through college. They are now in the range of their tall basketball teammates.

I reassure the family that Dione has "delayed constitutional short stature." I expect a delay in growth spurt and puberty. He should have an excellent spurt and puberty during his college years. I suggest that his family check his height in clinic or at home every few months. Dione's curve (the shape of the connected numbers on the growth chart) should run parallel to the average height curve.

DIAGNOSIS OF SHORT STATURE

The term "short stature" is used for children who are significantly shorter than their peers. When children have a routine health check, their heights and weights are plotted on the growth curve. This chart shows a growth path of the child's height and weight in relation to age. If the child's height is plotted on the 25th percentile line, it means that 75 percent of the children are taller than he or she is. This means that twenty-five out of a hundred children are shorter. A child is diagnosed as having short stature if the numbers plot at or below the 3rd percentile.

CAUSES OF SHORT STATURE

- *Familial short stature* is the most common basis for short stature in a child. A parent or both parents are short, but the rate of growth is normal. This is considered a genetic normal variant. If the cause of the short stature is familial, the bone age (a measure of maturity of the bones) is normal for age. The child will remain short as an adult.

- *Constitutional short stature* children will have normal adult height, but the process of gaining height will be prolonged. The child will be shorter than his or her peers but will catch up and pass the peers during college age. Often the child has a delayed age for puberty. The bone age matches the height, and the bones will mature in late adolescence. This cause has a genetic basis as an uncle, father, cousin, or sibling may report a similar progression. Dione and his family have constitutional short stature.
- *Idiopathic Short Stature* is a diagnosis of exclusion as the child is shorter than expected for parental height and has no known medical problems. There is currently no known cause for the height levels for these children. The bone age and weight are consistent for the height. There is current research being done to assess this cause.
- *Small for gestational age short stature* children were born prematurely and are thus smaller than their peers. It is rare for this shortness to persist; 90 percent will catch up with their peers.
- *Vitamin D deficiency short stature* involves a deficiency of vitamin D during childhood. This may cause a lack of growth and density of bones. This results in a bowing of the legs and thus a deficit in height.
- *Anemia short stature* can occur when decreased or pale red blood cells, often associated with iron deficiency, affect basic metabolism and thus decrease the production of proteins needed for growth.
- *Endocrine abnormality short stature* is seldom seen in children as they generally do not have abnormalities in the amounts of hormones in the body. However, there are some hormone (endocrine) imbalances that may cause short stature. These may be suggested by a physical exam showing short stature in an overweight child

or in cases of early or delayed puberty. These diagnoses must be verified by laboratory tests and bone age X-rays. The most common imbalance of hormones is hypothyroidism (low thyroid production). Rare is an overproduction of cortisol caused by overactive adrenals or by some medications. Decrease in growth hormone is also rare. The lack of this hormone results in significant short stature. Fortunately, the majority of cases of short stature caused by hormonal imbalance are treatable, especially if diagnosed in early childhood.

- *Genetic disease short stature* can result from rare diseases such as Turners (XO inheritance), trisomy 21 (Down syndrome), Russell Silver, Noonan syndrome and rare bone diseases all result in short stature. These are usually diagnosed in the infancy period.
- *Malnutrition short stature* can be found in children in many countries, including some developed countries, who do not receive adequate nutrients for standard growth.
- *Autoimmune disease short stature* is sometimes found in children with autoimmune diseases like lupus and juvenile arthritis, in which the body's immune system of white blood cells (lymphocytes) becomes confused and damages healthy cells. Muscles and joints may be involved, resulting in decreased growth.
- *Systemic* (involvement of many body parts) *disease short stature* occurs because most systemic diseases use a lot of the body's energy. Children with chronic diabetes type 1 or kidney or cardiac disease are often shorter than their peers. Chronic infections such as HIV or tuberculosis have a similar effect. Most of these children have poor appetites, which results in poor nutritional status. Cancer treatments using chemotherapy and/or radiation may cause a temporary cessation of growth.

- *Medications as cause of short stature* can be a negative side effect. Children with severe ADD may be treated for years with stimulants such as methamphetamines or other stimulants to increase focus. If used over years, the child may have a decrease in expected height. Steroids may be used for treatment of autoimmune diseases, some cancers, and asthma. If used for a short term, the child should not be affected. But months or years of use may result in less than expected height.

TREATMENT OF SHORT STATURE

As the causes of short stature are varied, the treatments are also varied. Low or high hormone levels are treated with hormonal medication and close observation. Dione's aunt, who has experience with sons with similar growth issues, asks that growth hormone shots be given. This hormone may increase his height by a spurt of growth, but it also increases his bone age and results in early puberty. Growth overall is sped up. His bones may seal over their growth ends at an early age, and growth will cease. He could end up shorter than initially forecast.

If a genetic cause is identified, the providers will know which organs should be assessed, and treatment can be started. Given at the right time, growth hormone has added height for some girls with Turners syndrome (female with XO gender chromosomes).

Children with chronic disease often resume their expected growth if the disease is controlled. Medications may be contributing to the short stature and need to be changed.

By far the causes of short stature are familial and constitutional. Patience and knowledge and acceptance are the best medicines!

Patience!

FOLLOW-UP FOR DIONE

Dione's family was reassured that he would probably remain the shortest boy in his class until late adolescence, when his growth spurt should push him up to his cousins' levels. Once he and his family looked at their relatives and listened to their stories of growth, they felt reassured and decided to just observe. After Dione and his family understood the different asthma medications, he had less episodes and did not need to use the steroid inhaler. He continues in excellent health and still hopes to be an NBA player and a team physician!

Go Warriors!

RESOURCES FOR FAMILIES

- Https://www.magicfoundation.org/Growth-Disorders/ Idiopathic-Short-Stature/ has information on idiopathic short stature.
- Https://www.emedicinehealth.com/short_stature_in_ children/article_em.htm has information regarding facts about short stature.

CHAPTER 11

Lucia: A Ten-Year-Old Whose Parents
Are Having Intense Custody Issues

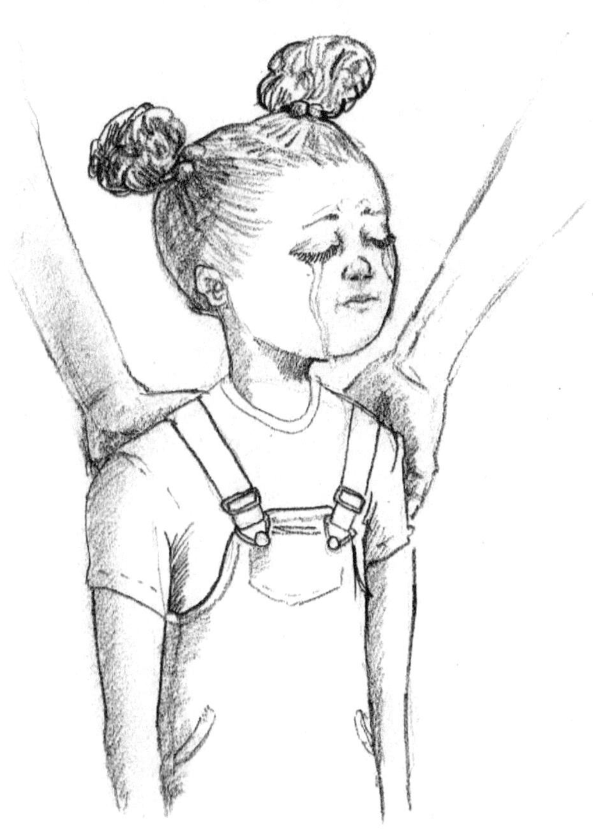

Lucia

LUCIA is a young girl who is experiencing intense reactions to her parents' impending divorce. A few weeks ago, her mother told Lucia and her siblings that she and Dad are separating. The kids knew there was trouble brewing as the criticisms, yelling, and slamming doors were increasing. Lucia's fourteen-year-old brother says he is happy that they are divorcing and that he will live with his dad. Her four-year-old sister seems confused and runs crying to her room whenever the subject comes up.

Lucia's father calls the clinic to ask for a referral for counseling as Lucia is acting oddly. He also asks for a letter for court stating that he is a good parent. The psychologist in clinic contacts the parents and advises they come for the first visit without Lucia. During the visit, the psychologist notes the hostility between the parents. They criticize each other and speak little regarding their daughters and son. The father says Lucia is refusing to speak to him when he calls and will not get in the car when he comes by to see them. He hears from his son that she cries a lot, refuses to eat some meals, and pretends she is sick. The mother says that Lucia is withdrawing from her family and friends. She cries when Dad comes by, has multiple wakings, wants to sleep with her mother, and shows disinterest in activities she used to love.

Lucia's father is worried because he and Lucia's mother are contesting custody issues in an upcoming court proceeding. Both want to be the custodial parent. Each says the other is unfit for parenting. The mother is upset about issues of discipline, diet, and the presence of other adults in the father's house. The father is upset about the constant conflict with the mother and

Lucia's emotional conflict. They say there are no drug, alcohol, or legal problems.

Lucia is withdrawn at the first meeting. After several visits, the psychologist learns that Lucia feels lonely, worried, and confused about taking sides. Because her mother is so upset, Lucia feels she needs to take care of her and comfort her during the sad and crying times. Lucia is unclear about custody issues and does not know what court will mean for her. She is fearful of moving, losing her friends, and attending a new school. She feels her brother and sister are happy as they will not hear the fighting if their parents are not together. She feels helpless and wants her mom and dad back together.

THE EFFECT OF DIVORCE ON CHILDREN

In the United States only 60 percent of children live with married parents. Fifty percent of marriages end in divorce. Often the following stressors affect the children.

- Living with a single parent
- Living in a different house or switching houses every few days
- Attending a new school
- Losing contact with friends
- Having less money as a second household is an added expense

Coparenting is sometimes not peaceful regarding living arrangements and decisions. The anger and hostility are often overwhelming for the children. Everyone in the family is experiencing loss and deep sadness. Emotions run the gambit from fear, confusion, shock to feelings of anger and guilt.

Children of all ages feel an internal guilt that they had some cause and effect on the separation. Younger children actually feel that a specific single behavior, like wetting the bed or breaking a vase, may have caused the split. Older children often become withdrawn and distance themselves from both parents. Although some children feel relief that the fighting may now end, most will express the wish that Mom and Dad were together. In some cases, divorce may be the best option for a family if conflict, fighting, or neglect becomes extreme, especially if there is violence or unsafe behaviors in the house.

As some parents show their pain and anger, they may turn to the child for comfort. This only increases the psychological trauma for the child. Some prepubertal or pubertal girls may feel that they need to act like a "wife" for Dad and do chores in his house. Some prepubertal or pubertal boys will feel like their Mom needs a "date" and will go to movies or watch TV to replace her partner. Some of these actions are obviously normal, but a continued pattern may be damaging.

Examples of the effects of divorce include:

- The affected child may have mood swings, being very needy verbally and physically or being very silent and withdrawn. These may occur with family or with friends.
- The child may exhibit anger or violent outbursts.
- Sleep problems of frequent waking and nightmares are common, especially if the child is moved to a new home.
- Problems may occur at school with acting out or withdrawing from friends and prior activities. Academic decline is common, usually caused by poor concentration.
- Physical signs, such as weight loss secondary to decreased appetite or stomachaches, often appear.
- In rare instances, a child may have serious reactions involving self-injury, such as cutting, or eating disorders.

Of course, none of the above may occur. Many parents understand the stress that divorce causes for their children. They are able to communicate honestly in a civil discourse. They will consider the practical aspects of divorce and try to make transitions as smooth as possible.

COMMUNICATING WITH CHILDREN ABOUT DIVORCE

- Parents must remain in a parenting role, listening carefully and seriously to their children's issues, but not allow the children to control the outcome.
- The children need some structure from the adults.
- Communication should be by both parents together, with calmness and respect and without conflict.
- There should be no delays or secrets in communication.
- Actions involving adultery, money, crimes, and so on do not need to be told in detail.
- Faults of either parent should not be a part of communication.
- Details should be simplified.
- Emphasis should be on the innocence of the children regarding the parents' choices. The divorce is between two adults. Children should be told they did nothing wrong to cause the divorce.
- Children should be reassured that the parents' love for them is always there.
- There should be acknowledgment of feelings of sadness and loss. Parents should show they understand their children's emotions without dwelling on their own loss.
- Both parents need to establish a consistent routine for living and visiting.
- Agreement regarding schedules and interactions is important. Changes should be minimal.

- Be aware of age differences in communication with the children.
- Agree on the issues regarding stepchildren and stepparents.
- Attempt to include relatives from both sides in the children's lives. Unless, of course, the relatives have their own problems that could affect the kids.
- Parents should try not to influence the children to take sides.
- Each parent should show respect for the other.

FOLLOW-UP FOR LUCIA

After several visits with her therapist, Lucia feels freer to talk to her parents about the divorce and what it means for her. In the first court hearing, the judge states there is no indication of neglect or potential danger to the children by either parent. Therefore, she rules that custody be split equally as possible between Mom and Dad for the girls. The girls decide to live with their mother during the school week, as she is better helping with homework, and weekends with Dad as he is more fun. The fourteen-year-old son chooses to live with his father but is advised to have regular visits with his mother. The custody issues regarding times and place for the five- and ten-year-old girls will be decided with an arbitrator and the parents. Family therapy is mandated.

After the final decisions were made with the parents and an arbitrator, Lucia felt more comfortable knowing the plans. She had a period of upset when a new stepmother and her children moved in with Dad. After the stepfamily was included in a few rough family therapy sessions, they all understood that the complex changes require respectful communication. As her mom progressed in her own therapy, she became socially involved, and Lucia felt less pressure. Lucia has begun to interact with friends and participate in activities. The siblings seem to have forged a pact that they will support each other.

I expect that there will be future ups and downs with this family, but they have experienced successful help in therapy and arbitration. Sometimes there is a maturity and openness in children who have been affected by divorce and learned the nuances of family structures. I sense the love and respect for others in this complex blended family.

Respect!

RESOURCES FOR FAMILIES

- Https://rainbows.org/services/divorce-support has a good discussion of issues and help finding support groups.
- Https://safeandsound.org/ has Kids Turn workshops with virtual meetings.

CHAPTER 12

Carlos: A Nine-Year-Old Boy Who Frequently Wets the Bed

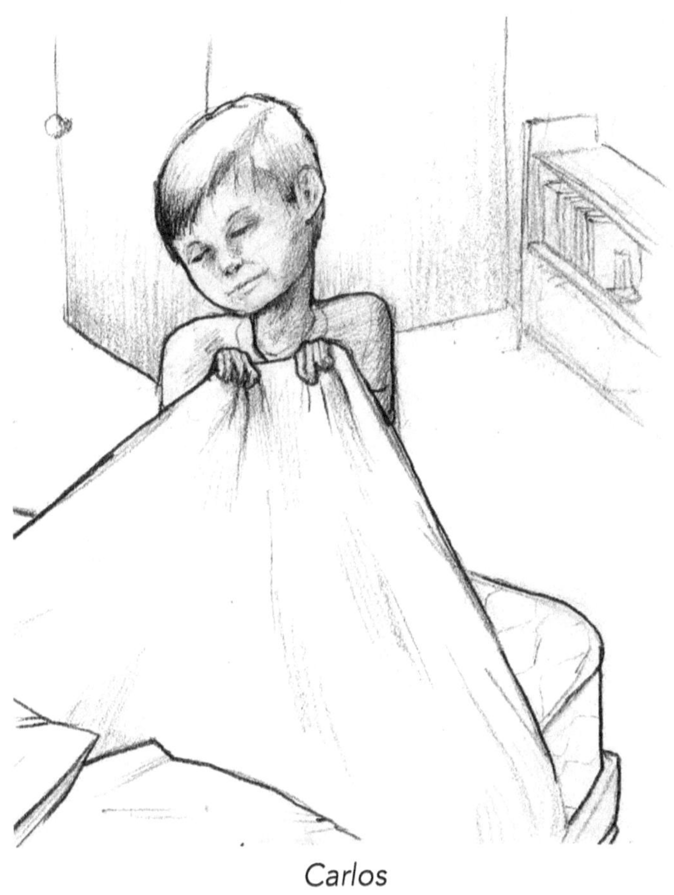

Carlos

CARLOS comes into my clinic with his mother, who is worried that he has kidney disease. "His aunt has polycystic kidneys, and his sister has frequent urinary tract infections. Carlos wets the bed every night." They had no problem potty training him for daytime urinating. They accepted the problem when he was a toddler and preschooler, but now it has become a hassle. They are exhausted in the morning with all the laundry. She tells me that she has tried to not let him drink anything before bed. It is difficult to wake him, so it is hard to take him to the bathroom around midnight, before she goes to bed. Carlos shares a bedroom with his older brother, who may wake when either Carlos or his mother is disruptive with the bedding. She says Carlos seems to be more and more upset about the problem. He even sometimes hides the sheets under the bed. Recently he has dragged his sheets and blankets to the laundry himself.

On further questioning about his symptoms, she mentions that Carlos never has accidents during the day, never has pain or bleeding with urination, and never has back pain. He explains that "I just don't wake up. Sometimes I feel afraid to fall asleep because I will wake up wet." When I ask how he feels about this, he says that he wishes he could go to camp or on overnights with friends. He always has to make up excuses and then feels guilty about lying and about missing time with his friends.

CARLOS'S CLINIC VISIT

I ask more detailed questions about how much Carlos drinks before bed. I ask how deep or well he sleeps and if he has pauses during sleep. I explain that wetting the bed usually happens in families. I ask the age of cessation of bed-wetting in family members. I am reassured when I learn the father's history of primary nocturnal enuresis (nighttime urination) until age eleven.

Carlos appears to be in excellent health with normal growth and blood pressure, both of which are usually abnormal if a child has kidney disease. His physical exam is normal with no physical signs of disease.

To make sure that Carlos does not have any of the rare problems that can affect the kidneys, we test his urine with a dipstick, which changes colors if there are any red or white blood cells, protein, glucose, abnormal pH (acid or base), or concentrated or diluted urine. Red blood cells or high protein may indicate something wrong with the filtering system of the kidneys. Red or white blood cells may indicate an infection. Glucose in the urine may indicate the child has diabetes. If pH is abnormal, the child may have an infection. If the urine is too diluted, the child may have diabetes insipidus, a hormonal problem, or the child may be drinking huge amounts of fluids. If the urine is too concentrated, the child may have dehydration from inadequate fluid intake. Fortunately, Carlos's urine is completely normal.

Because his aunt and sister have kidney problems, Carlos needs a renal (kidney) ultrasound to make sure the kidney system is anatomically normal. Rarely, a child may have unusual ureters, abnormal kidney or bladder shape, or cysts. Carlos's ultrasound is normal.

NOCTURNAL ENURESIS

If a child is over five and wetting the bed at night, and has a normal exam and normal laboratory tests, she or he may be diagnosed with *primary nocturnal enuresis*. This diagnosis is quite common in children over five and rarely an indication of a more severe medical problem. Primary nocturnal enuresis applies to the child who has never had control during the night but has urinary control during the daytime. *Secondary enuresis* applies to the child who once had control but now has new symptoms. This disorder is usually caused by an infection or by a change in lifestyle. The child will need further evaluation with lab tests and history.

Children are generally expected to be able to control their urination during the night by the age of five. However, bed wetting affects 20 percent of children who are five years old, but most children grow out of it with fewer being affected each year. There is a 44 percent risk that a child over five will wet the bed if one parent has a childhood memory of wetting the bed frequently, and a 77 percent risk if both parents wet the bed when they were young. Genetic studies have shown there is a genetic link to primary nocturnal enuresis.

HOW URINE IS MADE

The kidney is a filter system. As the blood flows through the two kidneys, unwanted chemicals from food, drugs, and normal body chemicals pass into the urine. Blood cells and important chemicals like protein, carbohydrates, and essential oils are held within the bloodstream. The urine then flows through tubes called ureters, which empties into the bladder where urine is held. When the time and place are right and the bladder is full, the urine will flow out the opening or sphincter into the outflow tube called the urethra. The urethra in boys is located in the penis. In girls, the urethra is just in front of the vaginal opening.

The timing, amount, and concentration of urination is controlled by chemicals in the brain. The pituitary gland produces a chemical called vasopressin that regulates our urination. When the bladder is full, nerves signal the brain. If it is not convenient to urinate at that time, the bladder opening, called the sphincter, tightens. If there is a good place and time to go, the brain will signal the sphincter to relax, and urine will flow out.

CAUSES OF NOCTURNAL ENURESIS

In rare cases children have an anatomic problem with the bladder being too small or the urethra opening is malformed, and the urine seeps out. Other children may have a delay in the nerve signals, and the sphincter will not tighten. These children with anatomic problems will lose urine both during the day and at night. Some children over-drink in the evenings, and the bladder will overflow. Other children will have a very deep sleep pattern and will not recognize the nerve signaling that the bladder is full, and the sphincter should remain tight. Children with extreme constipation may have a kinking of the sphincter, and urine will seep out.

A disease called diabetes insipidus, caused by a lack of vasopressin, results in very diluted and copious urine that overflows the bladder both in daytime and nighttime. Children with diabetes mellitus (diabetes type 1) have large amounts of sugar in the blood, and the kidneys increase urine production to try to balance the concentration of chemicals in the urine.

Some children do not want to use the bathrooms at their schools and may have overflow urination as the bladder cannot hold the urine for so long. A child may have a urinary tract infection with irritation of the bladder, which may cause some leaking. These illnesses cause leakage both during the day and at night.

Many children with ADD have primary nocturnal enuresis. It is speculated that these children may have differences in brain chemistry compared to other children and thus have either deep sleep or changes in their neurological signaling,

CAUSES OF BED-WETTING

- Over drinking of fluids
- Deep sleep patterns
- Sleep apnea
- Infection
- Diabetes insipidus
- Diabetes mellitus 1
- Nerve damage
- Severe constipation
- ADD

TREATMENT OF PRIMARY NOCTURNAL ENURESIS

The family is often exhausted but must refrain from shaming or blaming. For many children, treatment may be as simple as restricting fluids in the evening or having an adult wake the child and take her or him to the toilet before the adult goes to bed.

For children who are seven years old or older, a buzzer system may be helpful. These systems use a buzzer to wake the child when a small amount of fluid is detected by a sensor. They are effective for 30 to 60 percent of children. They help reinforce the waking impulse, which signals the bladder is full. This technique is more effective for the child nine to twelve years old. These buzzers are often sold in drugstores and are easy to locate on the internet.

Treatment with medications usually involves a synthetic hormone of vasopressin (DDAVP). This pill or nasal inhaler is taken at bedtime and is effective 60 percent of the time. DDAVP has minimal side effects. However, a common side effect is urinary retention, which is beneficial in these cases. Other unusual side effects are nausea, headaches, and muscle weakness.

In cases that are difficult to treat, we may order imipramine, a tricyclic antidepressant. The tricyclic drugs have the side effect of urinary retention, which is useful. Other side effects are blurred vision, dry mouth, nausea, and constipation or diarrhea. Neither of these medications will cure bed-wetting. They stop the symptoms during the time the child is on the treatment. Some children and families may decide to use vasopression only when a child is on a sleepover, camping trip, or family vacation.

FOLLOW-UP FOR CARLOS

I have learned it is important for families to be supportive and flexible with children who have this benign problem. Being aware of the importance of patience is more important than washing sheets! Telling the child that she or he is not alone is helpful. Carlos's dad is open to him regarding his own experience of stopping bed-wetting at age eleven. His parents plan to be very casual about laundry, using waterproof bed covers and teaching Carlos to help with his laundry so that he feels part of the solution.

Carlos begins to plan sleepovers and short-term camp sessions. He decides he can use a pair of sweatpants inside the sleeping bag that can be slipped off into the bag without anyone seeing it. Carlos's family is open to the use of medications on special nights or vacations if the enuresis persists.

I advise the family to use the bed-wetting event as a teaching moment to help the child appreciate the wonders of his or her body.

The human body is unique!

RESOURCES FOR FAMILIES

- Https://www.webmd.com/children/features/bedwetting-causes#1 is a site with explanations of bedwetting.
- Https://www.dailystrength.org/group/bedwetting is based on child-reader questions with blog-style answers.
- Https://www.mayoclinic.org/diseases-conditions/bed-wetting/symptoms-causes/syc-20366685 is a good source of general information on bed-wetting.

Acknowledgment

I could not have written this book without encouragement. Archway Publishers are excellent. Jason Shoemaker helped me with internet technology. Pablo Arroyo Ruiz, a noted artist, understood the kids I tried to portray. Numerous friends read passages and gave me honest reactions. My deepest thanks go to my sons and my spouse Emerson.